Epidermal Elegance: Understanding Your Skin and the Transformative Power of Professional Skincare

Table of Contents:

Chapter 1: Understanding the Skin Structure

Learn about the skin's anatomy, including the epidermis, dermis, and subcutaneous layers, and how they function to protect and maintain skin health. The skin is the largest organ in the human body and serves several essential functions. It consists of three primary layers: the epidermis, dermis, and subcutaneous tissue. The outermost layer, the epidermis, is a thin, protective barrier composed mainly of dead skin cells called keratinocytes. Beneath the epidermis lies the dermis, a thicker layer containing collagen, elastin, and other fibers that provide strength and elasticity to the skin. It also houses hair follicles, sweat glands, and sebaceous glands, which are responsible for producing sweat and sebum, respectively.

The dermis is crucial for the skin's overall health, as it plays a vital role in regulating body temperature and protecting against external pathogens. Deeper still is the subcutaneous tissue, comprising adipose cells that provide insulation and act as a shock absorber for the body.

The skin's complexity extends beyond its layers, with various specialized cells and structures that maintain its integrity and functionality. Melanocytes are responsible for producing melanin, the pigment that gives the skin its color and protects against harmful UV radiation. Langerhans cells are part of the immune system and defend against invading pathogens. Merkel cells are involved in the sense of touch and pressure.

Moreover, the skin's structure varies across different parts of the body, with variations in thickness, hair density, and the number of sweat glands. Understanding the skin's anatomy is crucial for medical professionals, as it aids in diagnosing and treating various skin conditions and diseases.

The skin's complex structure involves the epidermis, dermis, and subcutaneous tissue, along with a diverse array of specialized cells and structures. Its multifaceted functions encompass protection, temperature regulation, immunity, and sensory perception, making it an intricate and indispensable organ for the human body.

Chapter 2: Skin Types and Characteristics

Explore the different skin types (dry, oily, combination, and normal) and their unique characteristics, enabling you to tailor treatments to individual clients. Skin types and characteristics vary among individuals due to genetic, environmental, and hormonal factors. Broadly, there are five main skin types: normal, dry, oily, combination, and sensitive.

Normal skin is well-balanced, neither too oily nor too dry. It has a smooth texture, small pores, and a healthy glow.

Dry skin lacks sufficient moisture and may feel tight and rough. It is prone to flakiness, itchiness, and fine lines.

Oily skin, on the other hand, produces excess sebum, making it appear shiny and greasy. It is more prone to acne and enlarged pores.

Combination skin is a mix of oily and dry areas, often with an oily T-zone (forehead, nose, and chin) and drier cheeks.

Sensitive skin is easily irritated and may react to certain products or environmental factors, resulting in redness, itching, or burning sensations.

Each skin type requires different care and products. For normal skin, a balanced skincare routine with gentle cleansing and moisturizing is sufficient. Dry skin benefits from richer, hydrating products, while oily skin benefits from oil-free, non-comedogenic formulations.

Combination skin needs a targeted approach, with products suitable for both dry and oily areas. Sensitive skin demands mild, fragrance-free products, and patch testing new products is essential to avoid adverse reactions.

Understanding your skin type helps in tailoring a skincare regimen that addresses specific needs and maintains its health and appearance. Regular sun protection, hydration, and proper cleansing are essential for all skin types to maintain their optimal condition.

Chapter 3: The Science of Cleansing

Cleansing the skin is a crucial step in any skincare routine as it plays a pivotal role in maintaining skin health. The skin is the body's largest organ and consists of several layers, including the epidermis, dermis, and subcutaneous tissue. The epidermis, the outermost layer, serves as a protective barrier against environmental factors and pathogens. Regular cleansing helps to remove dirt, excess oil, makeup, and pollutants that accumulate on the skin's surface, preventing clogged pores and potential breakouts.

Estheticians play a significant role in providing deep cleansing treatments that target various skin concerns. Their expertise lies in using specialized products and techniques to effectively cleanse the skin's layers. During a deep cleansing session, an esthetician typically starts by analyzing the client's skin type and concerns. Estheticians then select appropriate products, such as cleansers, exfoliants, and masks, tailored to the client's needs. By using techniques like steam and gentle massage, estheticians help open up pores, allowing for a more thorough removal of impurities.

Delving deeper, the importance of deep cleansing goes beyond the surface layers. The dermis, situated beneath the epidermis, contains collagen, elastin fibers, blood vessels, and hair follicles. By properly cleansing the skin, these underlying structures can remain unburdened by the accumulation of dirt and debris. Additionally, regular deep cleansing supports the skin's natural cell turnover process, promoting the shedding of dead skin cells and aiding in the regeneration of new, healthier cells.

Estheticians utilize their knowledge and skills to perform extractions during deep cleansing, a process involving the removal of blackheads, whiteheads, and other impurities from clogged pores. This meticulous process requires professional expertise to avoid damaging the skin and causing inflammation. Estheticians might also employ advanced tools, such as ultrasonic devices or microdermabrasion, to enhance the efficacy of deep cleansing treatments and promote a smoother complexion.

In conclusion, deep cleansing is of paramount importance to all layers of the skin. It not only maintains the health of the skin's surface but also impacts the underlying structures and their functions. Estheticians play a crucial role in this process, utilizing their expertise to customize treatments, select appropriate products, and employ techniques that effectively cleanse the skin. By offering thorough cleansing, they contribute to the overall health and vitality of the skin, addressing concerns, promoting cellular regeneration, and aiding in the maintenance of a clear and radiant complexion.

Chapter 4: Exfoliation and Cellular Turnover

Cell turnover is a captivating and essential process that takes place in the skin, ensuring its continuous renewal and rejuvenation. The outermost layer of the skin, the epidermis, is composed of multiple layers of cells. As new cells are generated in the basal layer of the epidermis, they gradually move towards the surface. During this journey, older skin cells become compacted and eventually shed, making way for the fresher cells underneath.

This remarkable process of cell turnover has a profound impact on the skin's appearance and health. It promotes the removal of dead skin cells, which, if left unchecked, can lead to a dull and lackluster complexion. Moreover, regular cell turnover helps to minimize the appearance of fine lines, wrinkles, and age spots, contributing to a more youthful and vibrant skin texture.

Estheticians play a pivotal role in enhancing cell turnover through exfoliating treatments. Exfoliation involves the removal of dead skin cells from the skin's surface, encouraging the acceleration of the cell turnover process. Estheticians employ various exfoliation techniques, each catering to different skin types and concerns.

Physical exfoliation, also known as mechanical exfoliation, employs gentle abrasive materials or tools to physically slough away dead skin cells. This can include scrubs with fine particles, brushes, or microdermabrasion devices. Chemical exfoliation, on the other hand, involves the application of acids such as alpha hydroxy acids (AHAs) or beta hydroxy acids (BHAs) to dissolve the bonds between dead skin cells, facilitating their removal.

Estheticians assess each client's skin condition to determine the most suitable exfoliation method. They consider factors such as skin sensitivity, texture, sensitivity and any existing skin issues. By tailoring exfoliation treatments, estheticians help clients achieve optimal results without causing irritation or damage.

Regular exfoliation by an esthetician not only boosts cell turnover but also improves the efficacy of skincare products. By removing the barrier of dead skin cells, active ingredients can penetrate deeper into the skin, maximizing their benefits. This leads to better hydration, improved skin tone, and a smoother complexion.

In conclusion, the captivating process of cell turnover is a cornerstone of healthy skin. Estheticians contribute significantly to this process by offering expert exfoliating treatments that accelerate the shedding of dead skin cells, revealing fresher and more radiant skin. With their knowledge of various exfoliation techniques and their ability to tailor treatments to individual needs, estheticians play a vital role in helping clients achieve a rejuvenated and glowing complexion.

Body scrubs and detox treatments are also beneficial for skin health and appearance in several ways. Here's a breakdown:

Body Scrubs:

1. Exfoliation: The primary purpose of body scrubs is to exfoliate dead skin cells. By removing this top layer of dead skin, you're promoting smoother, more radiant skin.

2. Stimulates Skin Renewal: Exfoliation encourages the production of new skin cells, leading to more youthful-looking skin over time.

3. Cleansing: The ingredients in scrubs often help cleanse the skin, removing dirt and excess oils. This can prevent the occurrence of pimples, blackheads, and other blemishes.

4. Improved Blood Circulation: The massaging action when applying body scrubs can boost blood flow, aiding in the nourishment of skin cells. This results in healthier and more glowing skin.

5. Enhanced Product Absorption: Once the barrier of dead skin cells is removed, your skin can better absorb moisturizers or serums, making them more effective.

6. Relaxation: Many body scrubs contain essential oils which can offer aromatherapeutic benefits, aiding in relaxation and stress reduction. By reducing stress-related impediments and supporting overall health, in return relaxation indirectly promotes a healthy skin cell turnover rate which contributes to vibrant youthful complexion.

Body Detox Treatments:

1. Toxin Removal: Detox treatments are designed to draw out impurities from the skin. Ingredients like charcoal, clay, and certain salts can bind to dirt and pollutants, helping to remove them from the skin's surface.

2. Anti-Inflammation: Some detox treatments can reduce skin inflammation, which may help with conditions like acne or eczema.

3. Tightens the Skin: Ingredients such as clay can help tighten the skin, reducing the appearance of pores and providing a smoother skin texture.

4. Restores Skin Balance: By removing toxins and impurities, detox treatments can restore the natural balance of the skin, which is especially beneficial for those with oily or combination skin.

5. Hydration: Many detox treatments are formulated with moisturizing agents that help to hydrate the skin, leaving it soft and supple.

6. Nutrient Boost: Some detox products are enriched with vitamins and minerals that nourish the skin, promoting better skin health.

Both body scrubs and detox treatments can nourish and rejuvenate the skin by removing impurities, promoting circulation, and providing essential nutrients. It's essential, however, to choose products that are suitable for your skin type and to not over-exfoliate, as this can lead to irritation and sensitivity. Always follow the recommendations for the product and consult with a skin specialist (an esthetician) or dermatologist if you have concerns about your skin's health.

Chapter 5: The Power of Serums and Active Ingredients

Uncover the science behind potent serums and active ingredients, exploring their benefits for addressing specific skin concerns. Serums are potent skincare products formulated with high concentrations of active ingredients, designed to target specific skin concerns effectively. They come in various types, each with unique benefits and active ingredients.

1. Hydrating Serums: These serums are enriched with humectants like hyaluronic acid, glycerin, or panthenol that attract and retain moisture in the skin. They are beneficial for all skin types, particularly dry and dehydrated skin, as they provide intense hydration, improve skin elasticity, and plump up the skin's appearance.

2. Antioxidant Serums: Antioxidant-rich serums contain vitamins C and E, ferulic acid, green tea extract, and resveratrol, among others. These ingredients help neutralize free radicals, which are harmful molecules that contribute to premature aging and skin damage caused by UV radiation and environmental pollutants. Antioxidant serums are suitable for most skin types and can help reduce the signs of aging, improve skin texture, and protect against environmental stressors.

3. Brightening Serums: Brightening serums often contain ingredients like vitamin C, alpha arbutin, niacinamide, or kojic acid. These serums can help fade dark spots, hyperpigmentation, and uneven skin tone, making them ideal for those with sun damage or post-inflammatory hyperpigmentation. They can benefit most skin types but may require patch testing for sensitive skin.

4. Exfoliating Serums: Exfoliating serums contain alpha hydroxy acids (AHAs) or beta hydroxy acids (BHAs) that help to gently remove dead skin cells and unclog pores. AHAs, like glycolic acid, are water-soluble and work on the skin's surface, while BHAs, like salicylic acid, are oil-soluble and penetrate deeper into the pores, making them suitable for oily and acne-prone skin. Exfoliating serums can improve skin texture, reduce the appearance of fine lines, and promote a smoother complexion.

5. Soothing and Calming Serums: These serums often contain ingredients like chamomile, aloe vera, or centella asiatica extract, which have anti-inflammatory properties to soothe and calm irritated or sensitive skin. They are suitable for all skin types, particularly for those with redness or skin conditions like eczema or rosacea.

When choosing a serum, it's essential to consider individual skin type and concerns. For oily or acne-prone skin, a lightweight and non-comedogenic serum is preferable. Dry skin benefits from hydrating serums, while sensitive skin requires gentle and fragrance-free options. Always patch test new serums and introduce them gradually into your skincare routine.

In general, serums are powerful skincare products that target specific skin concerns with high concentrations of active ingredients. Hydrating, antioxidant, brightening, exfoliating, and soothing serums each offer unique benefits for different skin types and conditions. By incorporating the right serum into your skincare regimen, you can effectively address your specific skin concerns and achieve a healthier and more radiant complexion.

Chapter 6: Nourishing the Skin with Masks

Learn about different types of facial masks and their targeted benefits, from hydrating and soothing to purifying and brightening. Maintaining a healthy, nourishing routine for your skin is an integral part of a balanced beauty regimen. The skin, being the body's largest organ, serves as the first line of defense against various environmental factors and requires proper care to maintain its optimal function. A nourishing skin routine should encompass cleansing, toning, moisturizing, and sun protection, all tailored to your specific skin type. Skin types include oily, dry, combination, normal, and sensitive, and each has unique characteristics that require different care approaches. Dry skin may need more hydration and moisturizing, while oily skin needs oil control and non-comedogenic products. Regular cleansing is essential to prevent the accumulation of dead skin cells and excess oil, which can cause acne and other skin problems. Toning can help restore the skin's pH balance after cleansing, and moisturizing helps retain the skin's natural moisture.

Facial masks have been used for centuries in different cultures for their skin-enhancing properties. They can hydrate, nourish, cleanse, and rejuvenate the skin, depending on their ingredients and formulations. Clay masks, for instance, are great for oily skin types. They absorb excess oil and unclog pores, helping to prevent breakouts. Sheet masks, on the other hand, are ideal for dry skin as they help to hydrate and nourish the skin. They are typically soaked in a solution of hydrating ingredients and designed to lock in moisture. Peeling masks are good for combination skin, as they can address both dry and oily areas by exfoliating dead skin cells and promoting cell renewal. Cream masks, rich in oils and moisturizers, are best suited for dry or aging skin, providing it with the necessary nourishment and hydration. Gel masks are great for sensitive and sun-damaged skin, thanks to their soothing and cooling properties.

When it comes to key ingredients for different skin types, hyaluronic acid is a powerhouse ingredient for dry skin, as it can retain up to 1000 times its weight in water, providing intense hydration. Alpha and beta hydroxy acids (AHAs and BHAs), like glycolic acid, salicylic acid, and lactic acid, are excellent for oily and acne-prone skin. They exfoliate the skin, unclog pores, and reduce inflammation. Niacinamide is beneficial for all skin types, but particularly for those with acne or rosacea, as it helps to reduce redness, inflammation, and improve the skin's overall texture. Vitamin C, a potent antioxidant, can help brighten dull skin and reduce signs of aging, making it a great ingredient for mature skin. For sensitive skin, ingredients like aloe vera, chamomile, and green tea can help to soothe irritation and reduce inflammation.

Knowing your skin type and the right products to use is crucial for effective skincare. Each skin type has different needs that need to be addressed with suitable products and ingredients. With the right knowledge and routine, you can maintain your skin's health and vitality, improving its overall appearance and function. For optimal results, consulting with an esthetician can also be beneficial for providing specialized treatments tailored to your skin type.

Master the art of facial massage, understanding the benefits of lymphatic drainage and stimulating facial muscles for improved circulation. Facial massage is a widely practiced technique, heralded for its relaxing and rejuvenating properties. Originating from ancient Ayurvedic and Chinese medicine, the practice has been adopted worldwide for its potential to improve skin health. The art of facial massage goes beyond merely applying pressure to the skin; it's a delicate practice designed to stimulate blood flow, enhance lymphatic drainage, and promote collagen production. Besides the aesthetic benefits, facial massage also offers relaxation and stress relief, which contribute to overall well being. It's often performed using fingers, facial tools like jade rollers or gua sha stones, or even electronic devices.

The first step to an effective facial massage is preparation. Cleanse the skin to remove any makeup or dirt. Follow this with a suitable facial oil or serum to provide the necessary glide for the massage, minimizing friction that could potentially irritate the skin. While there are various types of facial massage techniques, they all center around gentle, upward movements that help defy the natural gravity pull. It's important to always use the ring finger for the delicate eye area, as it naturally has the least pressure.

One widely used facial massage technique is effleurage. It involves light, sweeping strokes made with the fingers or palms, usually at the beginning and end of a facial massage. Effleurage stimulates blood flow, warms up the muscles, and promotes relaxation. This method is often used to apply oil or cream and to conclude the massage, giving a general sense of wellbeing. Another method is petrissage, which uses kneading motions to lift and sculpt the facial muscles. This technique is particularly beneficial for aging skin, as it stimulates muscle memory and promotes skin elasticity.

A more intense technique is tapotement or percussion, which involves rapid, percussive tapping or slapping movements. This method is known to stimulate blood flow, enhance muscle tone, and revitalize the complexion. It can be a bit vigorous, so it's best to avoid using this technique on sensitive or inflamed skin. Friction, another technique, uses circular or transverse movements to generate heat, promoting circulation and encouraging cellular activity. This technique can help smooth wrinkles and fine lines, making the skin look fresher and younger.

The lymphatic drainage technique, sometimes referred to as the detoxifying massage, is particularly helpful for puffiness and fluid retention. It involves light, slow, rhythmic strokes aimed at stimulating the lymphatic system, helping to rid the body of toxins and reduce swelling. This method can be particularly beneficial for individuals with acne or rosacea, as it helps to clear the skin and reduce inflammation.

Lastly, there are facial massage techniques that specifically employ the use of tools. The jade roller, for instance, is a handheld tool often chilled before use to help with puffiness and inflammation. The roller is gently moved across the face, stimulating blood flow and promoting relaxation. The gua sha technique, originating from traditional Chinese medicine, uses a flat jade or rose quartz stone to scrape the skin gently. It's believed to promote energy flow, or "chi", and help with issues like tension, inflammation, and blood stagnation.

All in all, facial massage techniques have been employed for centuries to maintain skin health and radiance. With a wide variety of methods available, everyone can find a technique that best suits their needs and preferences.

Maderoterapia, also known as wood therapy, can be an effective technique not just for the body, but also for the face. Facial maderoterapia is a non-invasive massage technique that aims to improve the skin's appearance and health through the use of specially designed wooden tools. These tools come in different shapes and sizes, each serving a unique purpose depending on the area of the face being treated.

The facial maderoterapia process typically starts with a thorough cleansing of the face to ensure that the skin is clean and free of any makeup or impurities. A facial oil or serum may be applied to facilitate the smooth movement of the wooden tools on the skin and to provide additional skincare benefits. The specialist then uses the wooden tools to massage the face using upward and outward strokes, encouraging lymphatic drainage and blood circulation.

A variety of tools may be used during facial maderoterapia, each having a unique purpose. Smaller tools with smooth, rounded edges are used for the more delicate areas of the face, such as around the eyes and nose, to help reduce puffiness and dark circles. Larger tools with more surface area are used for the forehead, cheeks, and jawline to stimulate circulation, promote skin firmness, and help contour the face. There is even a roller tool, often with two or more balls, used to massage the skin, improve blood flow, and stimulate collagen production.

Regular facial maderoterapia can offer numerous benefits. It is known to help improve the skin's elasticity, reduce the appearance of fine lines and wrinkles, and give the skin a more youthful and radiant appearance. By stimulating blood flow, it brings more oxygen and nutrients to the skin cells, promoting healthier and brighter skin. Additionally, the massage can help stimulate lymphatic drainage, helping to eliminate toxins and reduce puffiness and inflammation.

It's important to note that while facial maderoterapia can yield positive results, consistency is key. A single session can provide immediate radiance and a feeling of relaxation, but regular sessions are recommended for lasting effects. It's also crucial to ensure that the therapy is performed by a trained professional to avoid any potential harm or discomfort. As with any skincare treatment, individuals should consult with their dermatologist or skincare professional to determine if facial maderoterapia is the right choice for their specific needs and skin type.

Gua Sha is an ancient Chinese healing technique that uses a smooth-edged tool, often made of jade, rose quartz, or stainless steel, to scrape or glide across the skin. The term "gua sha" translates to "scraping sands", referring to the redness or petechiae that may appear on the skin after a traditional gua sha treatment. When applied to the face, the technique is generally much gentler, aiming to stimulate circulation, encourage lymphatic drainage, and relax muscle tension, all of which can contribute to a brighter, firmer, and smoother complexion.

The process typically begins with cleansing the face and applying a facial oil to ensure the gua sha tool glides smoothly. The tool is then used to gently massage the face, starting from the center and moving outward and upward in a specific sequence. This might include the neck, chin, jawline, cheeks, under the eyes, eyebrows, and forehead. The pressure applied during facial gua sha is typically light to moderate, as the facial skin and muscles are delicate.

Apart from gua sha, other facial tools have gained popularity in skincare routines for their massaging and skin-enhancing benefits. Jade rollers, for example, are handheld tools often made of jade or rose quartz, with a larger roller on one end for broad areas like the forehead and cheeks, and a smaller roller on the other end for smaller areas like under the eyes. They are used to gently massage the face, promoting circulation and helping the skin to absorb products more effectively.

A relatively newer tool in the market is the facial roller massager or micro-needling roller. This tool features tiny needles that create micro-punctures in the skin when rolled across the surface. These punctures stimulate the skin's healing response, promoting the production of collagen and elastin, which can lead to a smoother and plumper skin appearance. However, this tool should be used with caution and proper hygiene as improper use can lead to skin irritation or infection.

Another tool gaining popularity is the facial cupping set. In facial cupping, small, specially designed cups are placed on the face to create suction, similar to traditional body cupping. This technique is thought to improve blood circulation, stimulate the skin, and enhance collagen production, leading to a healthier-looking complexion.

It's important to note that while these tools can contribute to skin health and appearance, they are not a replacement for a consistent skincare routine or professional medical advice. Proper technique and hygiene are crucial when using these tools to prevent skin damage or irritation. Always consult with a skincare professional or dermatologist to ensure these tools are suitable for your skin type and condition.

Chapter 8: Treating Acne

Delve into the complexities of acne, including its various types and factors contributing to breakouts, as well as effective treatment approaches. Acne is a common skin condition characterized by the occurrence of pimples, blackheads, whiteheads, and sometimes deeper lumps called cysts or nodules. While acne predominantly affects teenagers undergoing hormonal changes during puberty, it can affect individuals of all ages. Factors contributing to acne include excess oil production, clogged pores, bacteria, and inflammation. Furthermore, hormones called androgens increase in both boys and girls during puberty, enlarging the oil glands under the skin, leading to an overproduction of sebum, an oily substance that can clog pores and foster bacterial growth.

Acne can manifest in various forms and severities, ranging from mild, moderate to severe. Mild acne often presents as whiteheads or blackheads - small, non-inflamed blemishes that appear as tiny bumps on the skin surface. Moderate acne, on the other hand, is characterized by a higher number of whiteheads and blackheads, along with inflamed pimples that can be tender to touch. Severe acne typically presents as cystic acne, a deeper, more painful form of acne that often leads to scarring. Cystic acne requires immediate medical attention, as over-the-counter treatments are typically insufficient for this level of acne.

Treatment options for acne vary widely depending on its severity. Mild to moderate acne can often be controlled with good skincare habits and over-the-counter treatments. These can include topical treatments with active ingredients like salicylic acid, benzoyl peroxide, or retinoids, which help to unclog pores and reduce inflammation. Regularly washing the face, avoiding oil-based skincare products, and refraining from picking or squeezing blemishes can also help manage and prevent acne.

For moderate to severe acne, prescription medication may be necessary. These can include topical or oral antibiotics to combat bacteria, retinoids to prevent clogged pores, and hormonal treatments like birth control pills or spironolactone for women with hormone-related acne. In some cases, procedures like chemical peels, laser therapy, or drainage and extraction may be recommended to help clear up acne.

While acne is primarily driven by hormonal changes and genetic predisposition, certain lifestyle factors and medical conditions can exacerbate the problem. High levels of stress, a diet rich in refined carbohydrates and sugars, lack of sleep, and certain medications like corticosteroids can all contribute to acne. Medical conditions such as polycystic ovary syndrome (PCOS) and certain adrenal disorders can also cause acne due to an overproduction of androgens.

Acne can be a distressing condition, impacting one's self-esteem and quality of life. However, with an understanding of its causes and appropriate treatments, it can be effectively managed and treated. Always seek professional advice from a dermatologist to ensure you're receiving the right treatment for your specific type of acne and skin condition.

From a young age, I have fought a relentless battle with grade 4 acne, the most severe form of this skin condition. This type of acne, characterized by deep cysts, inflammation, and extensive skin damage, has posed not just physical challenges but mental and emotional ones as well. The myriad of skincare products and treatments I've tried in my quest to alleviate the symptoms often seemed like a never-ending cycle, with each attempt seeming more futile than the last. The physical discomfort, combined with the unpredictability of breakouts, made it feel like my skin was in a constant state of rebellion, relentlessly defying her attempts to restore its health and balance.

Every glance in the mirror was a stark reminder of my skin struggles. I noticed how the deep, painful cysts and extensive redness transformed the reflection I was accustomed to seeing. The physical manifestation of acne was only half the battle; the more challenging part was the mental toll it took on me. The relentless outbreaks seemed to be more than skin-deep, etching themselves onto my self-image, eroding my confidence bit by bit and it even spread to places like my shoulders, chest, and back. I yearned for the days when I could look at my reflection without the intrusive thoughts that often accompanied my gaze. The struggle with acne was not just about healing my skin, it was also about reclaiming my confidence and sense of self.

As a beauty professional, this struggle with severe acne felt particularly poignant. In an industry where I am used to enhancing the beauty of others, being unable to control my own skin condition is a bitter pill to swallow. Each day, as I painstakingly applied makeup to conceal my acne, I yearned for the freedom of a clear complexion. But it was through this battle that I found my strength. I began to understand that my value was not diminished by my skin condition and also had medical advice which has brought insight to the conclusion of my condition. My journey through this challenge was not easy, but it was a stark reminder that my self-worth was defined by more than just my appearance. Through my resilience and strength, I discovered a deeper beauty within myself that no skin condition could tarnish. I also remind myself that I went to school to become a skin therapist, like we try to express to our clients, "with time your skin will heal." I have to remember my skin is healing everyday, and the same for you, whatever your condition is.

Discover the causes of enlarged pores and effective treatments to minimize their appearance. Acne is a common skin condition that appears in various forms and degrees of severity. It occurs when your hair follicles become clogged with oil and dead skin cells. While it most commonly appears during puberty, it can affect individuals of all ages. Dermatologists often classify acne into four types or "grades" ranging from mild to severe. Recognizing the type of acne you have is crucial in determining the most effective treatment plan.

Grade 1, or mild acne, is characterized by occasional breakouts of whiteheads and blackheads. These are caused by the accumulation of oil and dead skin cells in hair follicles, which create plugs that appear as small bumps on the skin surface. In whiteheads, the pore is fully blocked, while in blackheads, the pore is partially open, allowing the plug to oxidize and turn black. Mild acne can often be managed with good skin care practices, including regular cleansing with a gentle, non-comedogenic cleanser, avoiding pore-clogging makeup and skincare products, and resisting the urge to pick or squeeze pimples, which can cause inflammation and scarring.

Grade 2, or moderate acne, typically includes frequent breakouts of whiteheads, blackheads, and pustules. Pustules are inflamed pimples filled with pus that often appear red at the base. Over-the-counter treatments containing salicylic acid or benzoyl peroxide can be helpful in reducing inflammation and unclogging pores. If these treatments aren't effective, a dermatologist may recommend prescription creams, gels, or lotions that contain retinoids, which are derivatives of vitamin A, known for their ability to unclog pores and reduce oil production.

Grade 3 acne, or moderately severe acne, involves numerous whiteheads, blackheads, pustules, and nodules, with evident inflammation. Nodules are larger, more painful pimples that are rooted deep within the skin. They may feel solid to the touch. Treating moderate to severe acne often requires a more aggressive approach, such as oral antibiotics to reduce inflammation and kill the bacteria that contribute to acne. In some cases, hormonal treatments may be prescribed, particularly for women who experience acne flares around their menstrual cycles.

Grade 4 acne, also known as severe or cystic acne, is characterized by numerous large, painful nodules and cysts, which are sac-like pockets of inflammatory material present deep within the skin. This type of acne can lead to significant scarring. It's typically treated with isotretinoin, a potent oral medication that can dramatically reduce sebum production, inflammation, and the presence of acne-causing bacteria. Isotretinoin treatment requires careful monitoring due to its potential side effects, and it's usually reserved for severe acne that hasn't responded to other treatments.

Regardless of the severity, managing acne often requires patience and consistency, as treatments may take several weeks or even months to show noticeable improvement. It's crucial to maintain a regular skincare routine, eat a balanced diet, manage stress, and get regular exercise, as these can all contribute to overall skin health. It's always wise to consult with a dermatologist or healthcare provider to discuss the best treatment options based on your specific needs and acne type.

Chapter 10: Managing Hyperpigmentation and Dark Spots

Explore the causes of hyperpigmentation and dark spots, and learn about advanced treatments like chemical peels and laser therapies. Hyperpigmentation is a common skin concern that refers to any darkening of the skin. It can present as localized dark spots, widespread discoloration, or patches of darker skin. This condition occurs when an excess of melanin, the pigment that gives skin its color, forms deposits in the skin. It can be triggered by various factors, including sun exposure, hormonal changes, injury to the skin, and certain medications.

There are different types of hyperpigmentation, each with its unique causes. Post-inflammatory hyperpigmentation (PIH), for instance, occurs following skin injury or inflammation such as acne, burns, or certain skin-care treatments. Melasma, another form of hyperpigmentation, is often linked to hormonal changes and is particularly common during pregnancy or among those taking oral contraceptives or hormone replacement therapy. Lastly, sunspots or age spots, known as solar lentigines, are caused by prolonged sun exposure over time.

Prevention is a key strategy in managing hyperpigmentation, and it begins with sun protection. Because UV radiation from the sun can trigger melanin production, it's essential to protect your skin by using a broad-spectrum sunscreen with an SPF of at least 30 every day, even when it's cloudy. Wearing protective clothing, such as hats and long-sleeved shirts, and seeking shade during peak sunlight hours can also help to protect your skin.

When it comes to treatment, several options can help lighten dark spots and even out skin tone. Over-the-counter products containing active ingredients like hydroquinone, retinoids, vitamin C, niacinamide, azelaic acid, kojic acid, and licorice root extract can help by disrupting the process of melanin production or speeding up the skin's natural exfoliation process to remove pigmented cells. These ingredients can be found in various products, such as creams, serums, and peels.

For persistent or widespread hyperpigmentation, more aggressive treatments may be necessary. These could include prescription-strength topical creams, chemical peels, laser therapy, microdermabrasion, or microneedling. These treatments work by removing the top layers of the skin to reduce the appearance of dark spots or by targeting the pigmented areas to break up the melanin deposits.

While these treatments can be effective, it's important to remember that results can take time, typically several weeks to months. Consistent use of treatment, as well as ongoing sun protection, is vital for success. In some cases, hyperpigmentation may be resistant to treatment, particularly in those with darker skin tones or in cases of deep or widespread pigmentation. It's also crucial to note that not every treatment is suitable for all skin types or conditions, so it's always best to consult with a dermatologist or skin care professional before starting a new treatment regimen for hyperpigmentation.

Chapter 11: Addressing Skin Sensitivity and Rosacea

Gain insights into sensitive skin and rosacea, discovering gentle and soothing treatments suitable for these conditions. Skin sensitivity is a common condition that affects numerous people worldwide, characterized by reactions such as redness, itchiness, or discomfort when the skin comes into contact with certain substances. These substances, known as triggers, can include beauty products, environmental factors like the sun or wind, and even specific foods. The key to managing skin sensitivity lies in both understanding its triggers and maintaining a solid skincare regimen.

Interestingly, skin sensitivity can be connected to a variety of factors. The epidermis, or outer layer of the skin, acts as a barrier against potential irritants. When this barrier is compromised, either due to genetic factors, aging, or environmental damage, skin sensitivity can result. Moreover, a weakened immune system, which often results from stress, can also contribute to skin sensitivity.

In managing sensitive skin, it's crucial to maintain a consistent skincare routine that focuses on strengthening the skin's barrier. Hydration plays a critical role in this. Regular use of a moisturizer that's suitable for your skin type can help to maintain the skin's natural barrier and prevent sensitivity. Furthermore, using mild, fragrance-free products can help to prevent irritation. Always remember to patch-test new products to ensure that they won't cause a reaction.

Rosacea, on the other hand, is a chronic, inflammatory skin condition that primarily affects the face. Symptoms can range from persistent redness and visible blood vessels to red, swollen bumps that resemble acne. While the exact cause of rosacea remains unknown, research suggests it could be due to a combination of hereditary and environmental factors.

The condition usually appears in individuals over 30 and is often mistaken for acne or other skin conditions. It's important to get a proper diagnosis from a dermatologist, as this can influence the kind of treatment you'll receive. For instance, certain acne treatments can actually worsen rosacea symptoms.

Managing rosacea typically involves a two-pronged approach: avoiding known triggers and following a prescribed treatment plan. Triggers can include anything from certain foods and drinks to emotional stress and weather conditions. Keeping a diary can be useful in identifying these triggers.

Treatment options for rosacea range from topical creams and oral medications to laser therapy. While there's no cure for rosacea, these treatments can help control and reduce the signs and symptoms. Remember, each person with rosacea is unique, so what works for one person might not work for another. This is why it's essential to work closely with a dermatologist to find a treatment plan that works best for you.

Chapter 12: Sun Protection and Anti-Aging

Examine the crucial role of sun protection in preventing premature aging and explore anti-aging treatments to minimize fine lines and wrinkles. Sun protection is more than just a step in your daily skincare routine; it's an essential measure for overall skin health. Sun exposure is known to cause a vast majority of skin aging signs, including wrinkles, discoloration, and loss of elasticity. It's not just about avoiding the sun at its peak; it's about integrating sun protection into your daily life.

The sun emits two types of harmful rays - UVA and UVB. UVA rays penetrate deep into the skin and can lead to premature aging, also known as photoaging, while UVB rays can cause sunburn and play a key role in developing skin cancer. This is why dermatologists recommend using a broad-spectrum sunscreen, which protects against both UVA and UVB rays.

It's not enough to just apply sunscreen; it's crucial to apply it correctly and consistently. Aim for at least an SPF 30 and apply a generous amount to all exposed skin about 15 minutes before heading outdoors. Remember, sunscreen isn't just for sunny days. Even on cloudy days, up to 80% of the sun's harmful UV rays can penetrate your skin.

Even the most dedicated sunscreen application is not enough to fully protect your skin. Wearing protective clothing, such as a wide-brimmed hat, and seeking shade during the sun's peak hours can provide additional protection. Don't forget about sunglasses; they not only protect your eyes but also the sensitive skin around them.

On the other hand, anti-aging skincare is about more than just preventing wrinkles. It involves understanding the skin's aging process and how to slow it down. As we age, our skin naturally loses collagen and elastin, two proteins that keep our skin firm and smooth. The loss of these proteins leads to the formation of wrinkles and sagging skin.

A key part of any anti-aging routine is moisture. Hydrated skin looks plumper, minimizing the appearance of fine lines and wrinkles. This means not only using a good quality moisturizer but also drinking plenty of water and avoiding dehydrating habits like smoking and excessive alcohol consumption.

Incorporating products with anti-aging ingredients into your skincare routine can also make a significant difference. Retinoids, derivatives of vitamin A, are widely considered the gold standard in anti-aging skincare. They work by promoting cell turnover, which helps to smooth wrinkles and improve skin texture.

Antioxidants, such as vitamin C, are another cornerstone of anti-aging skincare. They combat free radicals, unstable molecules that can cause damage to the skin cells and accelerate the aging process. Using a vitamin C serum in the morning can help protect your skin from free radical damage throughout the day.

Lastly, remember that healthy skin starts from within. A balanced diet rich in fruits, vegetables, lean proteins, and healthy fats can provide your skin with the nutrients it needs to stay healthy and youthful. Regular exercise can also improve circulation, which helps to keep your skin looking vibrant. It's a comprehensive approach that requires consistency, but the results are well worth it.

Chapter 13: The Importance of Hydration

Understand the significance of skin hydration and how to effectively hydrate and lock in moisture for plump and supple skin. "Water is the driving force of all nature", as Leonardo da Vinci once stated, and nowhere is this more apparent than in the human body. Hydration plays a critical role in maintaining health, influencing everything from cognitive function and physical performance to skincare and digestion. Drinking enough water each day is crucial for many reasons and forms an integral part of our well-being.

To begin with, hydration is key to supporting the optimal functioning of our bodily systems. The human body is around 60% water, and every single cell, tissue, and organ needs it to function properly. Water acts as a building block, a solvent for chemical reactions, and a transport material for nutrients and waste. In the brain, it acts as a shock absorber and plays a significant role in producing hormones and neurotransmitters.

In terms of physical performance, proper hydration is a game-changer. It aids in maintaining body temperature, lubricating joints, and facilitating muscle function. Dehydration can negatively impact physical performance, causing fatigue, reducing endurance, and lowering strength. On the other hand, staying well-hydrated enhances cardiovascular health, cools the body, and aids muscle recovery.

On the skincare front, hydration is synonymous with a healthy glow. Adequate hydration helps to keep the skin plump, elastic, and resilient. Water is essential to maintain the optimum skin moisture and deliver essential nutrients to the skin cells. It replenishes the skin tissue and increases its elasticity, which can help delay the appearance of signs of aging such as wrinkles and fine lines.

Further, hydration aids digestion and helps maintain a healthy weight. Water aids in the digestion of food and the absorption of nutrients, ensuring that the body gets the most nutritional value from your meals. It also helps you feel full, which can aid in weight management by reducing overeating. Additionally, proper hydration can prevent or alleviate constipation by keeping the stool soft and easy to pass.

The benefits of staying hydrated also extend to our mental health. Dehydration can affect your mood and cognitive functions, leading to symptoms such as irritability, confusion, or fatigue. A well-hydrated brain is well-equipped to manage stress, can think more clearly, and maintain a balanced mood.

While the amount of water each person needs can vary based on factors like age, sex, weight, and activity level, a general guideline is to aim for eight 8-ounce glasses, which equals about 2 liters, or half a gallon a day. This is the 8x8 rule and is easy to remember. Remember that other fluids and foods with high water content also contribute to your daily water intake. Ensuring you get enough hydration is a small step with a big impact, a simple habit that can boost your health and vitality.

Chapter 14: Building a Skincare Routine

Guide clients in developing a personalized skincare routine, incorporating proper cleansing, exfoliation, hydration, and sun protection. A skincare routine is like a health routine for your skin, the body's largest organ. Building an effective skincare regimen is crucial not only for immediate aesthetic results but also for the long-term health and appearance of your skin. It helps prevent skin issues, keep your skin in good condition, and combat the effects of aging. A regular skincare routine can help you to identify your skin type and understand its specific needs.

The first step to building a skincare routine is to understand your skin type. Is it oily, dry, combination, or sensitive? This forms the foundation of your routine, as it determines what kinds of products you'll need. The skincare industry offers a wide variety of products, and knowing your skin type helps narrow down the options, making it less overwhelming and more effective.

A basic skincare routine consists of three key steps: cleansing, toning, and moisturizing. Cleansing removes dirt, oil, and makeup from your skin. A good cleanser leaves your skin feeling clean but not stripped of its natural oils. Toning is the second step. A toner helps remove any residual dirt or makeup left after cleansing and preps the skin for the next step. It restores the pH balance of the skin and tightens the pores. The third step is moisturizing. A moisturizer locks in hydration, helps strengthen your skin's protective barrier, and keeps your skin soft and smooth.

A consistent skincare routine not only affects the outward appearance of your skin but also its overall health. Regular cleansing prevents the build-up of oils and dirt that can lead to breakouts and inflammation. Likewise, consistent use of a moisturizer can improve your skin's hydration levels and help strengthen the skin's barrier function, leading to more resilient skin over time.

Beyond the basic steps, incorporating additional treatments like exfoliators, serums, and masks can further enhance your skincare routine. Exfoliation helps to remove dead skin cells that can clog pores and lead to a dull complexion. Serums deliver a high concentration of active ingredients to target specific skin concerns like fine lines, dark spots, or dehydration. Masks provide an extra boost of nourishment and are tailored to specific skin needs.

Sunscreen, a non-negotiable part of your daily routine, should be applied every morning. It protects your skin from harmful UV rays that can lead to premature aging and skin cancer. Regardless of whether it's sunny or cloudy, harmful UV rays can still penetrate your skin, making daily sunscreen use vital for maintaining skin health.

The importance of a skincare routine extends beyond the physical. The practice of taking care of your skin can also provide a moment of relaxation and self-care in your daily routine. It can serve as an opportunity to check in with yourself and take a few moments just for you. Remember, the most effective routine is the one you enjoy and stick to.

Chapter 15: Prioritize Skincare with Self-Care

The concept of self-care goes beyond merely caring for one's physical body. It encompasses the pursuit of activities that contribute to overall well-being, including mental, emotional, and spiritual health. Skin care, while commonly perceived as a simple act of hygiene, can be a powerful tool in the realm of self-care. This is due to its potential to encourage mindfulness, routine, and a sense of control, all while promoting skin health.

Skin care can provide a sense of routine and structure. Whether your routine involves only a few basic steps or a more comprehensive regimen, the consistent practice can create a soothing, predictable rhythm in your day. This can be particularly beneficial during times of stress or uncertainty, when maintaining a routine can help create a sense of normalcy and stability.

However, the very act of skin care can be a form of mindfulness. Mindfulness involves staying present and engaged in the current moment. When applying products, focus on the sensation of the product on your skin, the aroma of the ingredients, and the feeling of your fingers against your face. This can help create a calming, meditative moment, allowing a brief respite from the demands of the day.

Taking care of your skin can also be an act of self-empowerment. By choosing to engage in a skincare routine, you are making a decision to care for yourself. This act of choosing can foster a sense of control and self-efficacy, which can be particularly beneficial during stressful periods when many aspects of life may seem out of control.

Besides these psychological benefits, a good skincare routine is fundamental for maintaining healthy skin. Cleanse regularly to remove dirt, oil, and pollutants, exfoliate to remove dead skin cells, hydrate with a good moisturizer, and always apply sunscreen to protect against harmful UV rays. This helps to keep your skin healthy, vibrant, and can prevent skin conditions or premature aging.

Nutrition and hydration are also integral to skin health, reflecting the intersection of skincare with broader self-care practices. A balanced diet rich in vitamins, minerals, and antioxidants can help protect and repair skin. Hydration, both through drinking plenty of water and using hydrating skincare products, is vital to maintain skin's elasticity and prevent dryness or flakiness.

A skincare routine provides more than just a clear complexion—it contributes to a broader self-care practice that nurtures the mind and body. By prioritizing skincare, you prioritize yourself, creating space for wellness, calm, and self-affirmation. This highlights the importance of viewing skincare as not just an obligation or a luxury, but as a valuable component of a holistic self-care routine.

Chapter 16: Holistic Skincare and Nutrition

Explore the connection between skincare and nutrition, recommending skin-boosting foods and supplements for overall well-being. Holistic skincare is a growing approach to skin health, emphasizing the connection between overall health and the skin's appearance. This approach views the skin as a reflection of the body's internal state, taking into account factors like diet, lifestyle, and emotional wellbeing. It's about caring for the skin from the inside out, focusing on overall wellness as the foundation for healthy, vibrant skin.

At the core of holistic skincare is the understanding that our skin is affected by more than just the products we apply to it. Environmental factors, stress levels, sleep patterns, and, most notably, our diets all play a significant role. Our skin is the body's largest organ, and like any other organ, it needs a range of nutrients to function optimally.

To take a holistic approach to skincare, it's important to recognize the role of nutrition. The food we consume has a direct impact on our skin's health. For instance, eating a diet rich in antioxidants can help protect the skin from damage caused by free radicals, unstable molecules that can harm the structural integrity of the skin cells. These antioxidants can be found in a variety of fruits and vegetables, particularly those with vibrant colors.

Omega-3 fatty acids, found in fish and flaxseeds, are another essential component of a skin-healthy diet. They have anti-inflammatory properties, which can help soothe skin conditions like eczema and psoriasis. They also support the skin's barrier function, helping to lock in moisture and keep out irritants.

Hydration, as we've touched on before, is vital for skin health. Drinking enough water supports the skin's elasticity and can help prevent dryness and flaking. However, it's not just about drinking water; it's also about consuming foods with high water content, like cucumbers, watermelon, and berries.

In holistic skincare, we also recognize the impact of lifestyle factors on our skin. Regular physical activity, for instance, can increase blood flow, helping to nourish skin cells by carrying oxygen and nutrients to them. It also helps to flush cellular debris out of the system, essentially cleansing the skin from the inside out.

The holistic approach also considers the mind-skin connection. Chronic stress can cause inflammation in the body, leading to issues like acne and accelerated aging. Implementing stress-reducing practices such as yoga, meditation, or simple breathing exercises can help to manage stress levels and, by extension, support skin health.

Holistic skincare represents a shift away from quick fixes and towards sustainable, long-term skin health. It's a comprehensive approach that requires consistency and commitment but can lead to improved skin and overall health. Understanding that the skin is an outward reflection of our internal health allows us to care for it in a more intentional and effective way.

Chapter 17: Understanding Eczema and Dermatitis

Learn about eczema and dermatitis, their triggers, and gentle treatments to soothe and alleviate symptoms. Eczema and dermatitis are terms often used interchangeably to describe a group of conditions that cause the skin to become red, itchy, and inflamed. Despite sharing similar symptoms, they are, in fact, different types of skin conditions that can have various causes and treatments. Understanding the differences and similarities between these conditions can aid in managing their symptoms and maintaining skin health.

Eczema is a chronic inflammatory skin condition characterized by dry, itchy patches on the skin. The most common type of eczema is atopic dermatitis. While the exact cause of eczema is unknown, it is believed to be linked to an overactive immune system response to irritants. Eczema often flares up in response to certain triggers, which can vary widely among individuals but may include harsh soaps or detergents, certain fabrics, fragrances, and even weather conditions.

Atopic dermatitis often runs in families, suggesting a genetic component, and is often seen in those with a family history of allergies, hay fever, or asthma. While it can occur at any age, it's most common in children, and many outgrow the condition or see a significant reduction in symptoms as they get older.

Maintaining a regular skin care routine can help manage eczema symptoms. This typically includes bathing with a gentle, fragrance-free cleanser, followed by the application of a moisturizer to lock in hydration. During a flare-up, over-the-counter creams and ointments that contain the steroid hydrocortisone can help reduce inflammation and relieve itching.

Dermatitis, on the other hand, is a general term that describes skin irritation. There are several types of dermatitis, each with different causes. Contact dermatitis, for instance, is caused by direct contact with certain substances. It can be either irritant contact dermatitis, caused by substances like bleach or soaps, or allergic contact dermatitis, where an allergic reaction occurs after skin comes into contact with an allergen, such as nickel or poison ivy.

Seborrheic dermatitis is another common type, which appears as red skin, scaly patches, and dandruff, most often on the scalp. It's thought to be related to the Malassezia fungus, which is normally present on the skin's surface, but can overgrow in certain conditions, leading to dermatitis.

Treatment for dermatitis depends on the type and severity. For contact dermatitis, the best treatment is to identify and avoid the substances causing the reaction. Over-the-counter creams and ointments can also help to reduce inflammation and itching. For seborrheic dermatitis, antifungal treatments and medicated shampoos can be effective.

Understanding the specific type and cause of your skin condition is crucial for effective treatment. While eczema and dermatitis can cause discomfort and stress, they are often manageable with the right care. Working with a healthcare provider or a dermatologist can help determine the best approach to managing these conditions. A comprehensive skincare routine, combined with lifestyle factors such as a balanced diet and stress management, can contribute significantly to maintaining skin health.

Chapter 18: Targeting Fine Lines and Wrinkles

Delve into the science of aging, understanding the causes of fine lines and wrinkles, and explore treatments like retinol and dermal fillers. Fine lines and wrinkles are natural signs of aging that reflect the lifelong journey our skin has undertaken. They occur due to the gradual loss of collagen and elastin in the skin, substances that provide our skin with structure and elasticity. Environmental factors, such as sun exposure and lifestyle choices like smoking or poor nutrition, can also contribute to their formation. While they are a normal part of aging, understanding what causes them can help us adopt practices to mitigate their appearance and maintain youthful-looking skin.

The appearance of fine lines is typically the first sign of skin aging. These shallow lines often occur in areas where the skin naturally folds during facial expressions, such as around the eyes and mouth. They're usually minor and can be hard to see initially, but over time, without proper care, they can develop into deeper creases, or wrinkles.

Wrinkles are deeper folds in the skin that are more noticeable than fine lines. They often appear on parts of the body that get the most sun exposure, including the face, neck, backs of the hands, and tops of the forearms. They can also be caused by factors like facial muscle contractions or gravity over time.

Sun protection is a crucial factor in preventing and minimizing the appearance of fine lines and wrinkles. UV radiation accelerates the natural aging process, breaking down the skin's collagen and elastin fibers, which results in wrinkling and sagging of the skin. Using a broad-spectrum sunscreen, wearing protective clothing, and seeking shade can significantly reduce sun damage.

Skincare can also play a significant role in managing fine lines and wrinkles. Regular use of moisturizer can help the skin appear plumper and minimize the appearance of wrinkles. Retinoids, derivatives of vitamin A, are another potent tool in the fight against aging. They can stimulate the production of new skin cells and encourage the formation of new collagen.

In addition to topical treatments, certain in-office procedures can help reduce the appearance of fine lines and wrinkles. These include chemical peels, dermabrasion, and laser resurfacing, which remove the outer layer of skin to reveal new, smoother skin underneath. Injections of botulinum toxin (Botox) or fillers can also help smooth out wrinkles and fine lines.

Lifestyle changes, like maintaining a healthy diet rich in antioxidants, staying well-hydrated, getting enough sleep, and not smoking, can also contribute significantly to minimizing the appearance of fine lines and wrinkles. These healthy habits can help to preserve the skin's natural elasticity and slow down the aging process.

In essence, fine lines and wrinkles are a natural part of life and aging. However, with a consistent skincare regimen, sun protection, and healthy lifestyle choices, it's possible to delay their onset and lessen their appearance. Consulting with a dermatologist or skincare professional can provide personalized guidance on the best strategies for your specific skin needs.

Dermal fillers are a popular cosmetic treatment used to minimize the appearance of fine lines and wrinkles, and to restore volume and fullness to the skin. As we age, our skin naturally loses subcutaneous fat, and the facial muscles start working closer to the skin's surface, which makes lines and wrinkles more apparent. Dermal fillers can help to fill in these lines and add volume, giving the face a more youthful appearance.

There are several types of dermal fillers, each designed to treat different signs of aging or other cosmetic issues. The most common type of filler is hyaluronic acid, a substance that is naturally produced by the body. Hyaluronic acid fillers can add volume and smoothness to the skin, reducing the appearance of lines and wrinkles. They can also stimulate the production of collagen, a protein that helps maintain the skin's elasticity.

Another type of filler is poly-L-lactic acid, a biocompatible, biodegradable substance that helps to replace lost collagen. This type of filler is used to treat deep facial wrinkles and to add volume to thinning areas of the face. It works gradually over a series of treatments, typically over a few months, and can last for up to two years.

Calcium hydroxylapatite is a substance found naturally in our bones. When used as a filler, it is suspended in a gel-like solution and can provide immediate results. It is typically used for deeper lines and wrinkles and to enhance fullness in areas like the cheeks and jawline. The effects of calcium hydroxylapatite fillers can last up to 12 months or longer.

One key advantage of dermal fillers is that they are minimally invasive and have a relatively short recovery time. The procedure itself usually takes less than an hour, and most people can return to their regular activities immediately afterward. However, some mild side effects can occur, such as redness, swelling, and bruising at the injection site.

Despite the benefits of dermal fillers, it's crucial to remember that they are a medical procedure and should be performed by a qualified healthcare professional. When considering dermal fillers, you should discuss your medical history, aesthetic goals, and expectations with your provider to determine the best treatment plan for you.

In summary, dermal fillers can be an effective way to address signs of aging, including fine lines and wrinkles. They offer a minimally invasive solution for those seeking to restore volume and smoothness to their skin. As with any cosmetic procedure, it's essential to understand the process, risks, and benefits to make an informed decision that best suits your individual needs and aesthetic goals.

Chapter 19: Dealing with Under-Eye Circles and Puffiness

Explore the causes of under-eye circles and puffiness, as well as treatments such as eye creams and lymphatic drainage massages. Under-eye circles and puffiness can give you a tired appearance, even when you're well-rested. These issues can be caused by various factors, including age, allergies, sleep deprivation, and individual genetics. Understanding the underlying cause is the first step in effectively addressing under-eye circles and puffiness.

Dark circles often result from the thinning of the skin and loss of fat and collagen, common as we age. This thinning can make the reddish-blue blood vessels under your eyes more noticeable. Allergies can also contribute to dark circles. When you have an allergic reaction, your body releases histamines, causing an inflammatory response that can lead to puffiness and dark circles. Additionally, lack of sleep or excessive sleep can exacerbate the appearance of dark circles.

To minimize the appearance of dark circles, adequate sleep is paramount. Aim for 7-9 hours per night, and consider elevating your head with an extra pillow, which can prevent fluid from pooling under your eyes. Incorporating a vitamin C serum into your skincare routine can also help. Vitamin C is a potent antioxidant that can lighten skin, boost collagen production, and counteract the damaging effects of UV exposure. For stubborn dark circles, retinoid creams can stimulate collagen production, making the skin under the eyes thicker and less translucent, thus hiding the dark blood vessels.

Under-eye puffiness or bags are often due to the accumulation of fluids and can be influenced by diet, especially the consumption of salty foods that can cause water retention. Aging also plays a role, as the tissues and muscles supporting your eyelids weaken, causing fat to migrate to the lower eyelids, creating a puffy appearance.

To combat puffiness, consider a cold compress or cooling eye masks, which can constrict blood vessels and reduce swelling. Reducing dietary salt and alcohol, both of which can cause fluid retention, may also help reduce puffiness. Incorporating a gentle eye massage into your skincare routine can stimulate blood circulation and aid in the draining of excess fluid.

Certain skincare products can also be beneficial. Eye creams with ingredients like caffeine can constrict blood vessels and reduce puffiness, while creams containing hyaluronic acid can hydrate and plump the skin, reducing the appearance of fine lines and sunken eyes. Retinoids can help by increasing cell turnover and collagen production.

For those with persistent under-eye circles and puffiness that don't respond to lifestyle or skincare changes, cosmetic treatments might be an option. Treatments such as filler injections or laser therapy can minimize the appearance of under-eye circles, while blepharoplasty, a type of eyelid surgery, can remove excess fat and skin to reduce puffiness. As with any medical procedure, these treatments should be discussed with a qualified healthcare professional to assess suitability and potential risks.

Dealing with under-eye circles and puffiness can often be frustrating, but with a multi-faceted approach that includes good sleep habits, a healthy diet, proper skincare routine, and potentially professional treatments, these common concerns can be effectively managed. It's always best to consult with a skincare professional or dermatologist to guide your approach based on your unique needs.

Chapter 20: Skincare for Men

Tailor skincare advice specifically for men, understanding their unique skin concerns and preferences. While skin care has often been marketed as predominantly a concern for women, the reality is that men's skin needs attention and care just as much. Factors such as daily shaving, exposure to the elements, and the general composition of male skin, which tends to be thicker and oilier than female skin, all call for a well-designed skincare routine for men.

The cornerstone of any skincare routine, regardless of gender, is cleansing. For men, cleansing not only removes dirt, excess oil, and impurities from the surface of the skin but can also help to prepare the skin for a smoother shaving experience. Opting for a gentle, non-comedogenic cleanser that doesn't strip the skin of its natural oils is crucial. Cleansing should be done twice a day, in the morning and at night, to keep the skin clean and healthy.

Exfoliation is another critical step, especially for men who shave regularly. Regular exfoliation can help prevent ingrown hairs by removing dead skin cells that can clog hair follicles. It can also help to smooth the skin's texture, brighten the complexion, and allow for better absorption of other skincare products. However, because exfoliation can be quite powerful, it's recommended to limit this practice to once or twice a week to avoid over-exfoliation, which can lead to skin irritation and dryness.

Shaving can be tough on the skin, causing irritation, dryness, and even minor cuts. Using a high-quality shaving cream or gel can provide a protective layer between the skin and the razor, reducing the risk of irritation. Following up with an alcohol-free aftershave or balm can help soothe and hydrate the skin post-shave. It's also worth mentioning the importance of maintaining clean, sharp razors to ensure a clean shave and minimize skin irritation.

Just like for women, moisturizing is an essential step in men's skincare. A good moisturizer can help to replenish hydration, seal in moisture, and leave the skin looking healthy and vibrant. Men with oilier skin might prefer a lightweight, oil-free moisturizer, while those with dry or sensitive skin may benefit from a more nourishing formula.

Sun protection is non-negotiable, regardless of gender. Men should incorporate a broad-spectrum sunscreen with at least an SPF of 30 into their daily routine. Sunscreen not only protects the skin from harmful UV rays that can cause premature aging and skin cancer, but it can also help prevent hyperpigmentation and uneven skin tone.

Lastly, addressing specific skin concerns is also important. This could involve using a retinoid for fine lines and wrinkles, a targeted spot treatment for acne, or a dark spot corrector for hyperpigmentation. Men can also benefit from regular visits to a dermatologist or skin care professional for personalized advice and treatment options.

In essence, while men's skincare needs can differ slightly from women's, the basics remain the same: cleanse, exfoliate, moisturize, protect, and treat. Building a skincare routine doesn't have to be complicated or time-consuming. Even a few simple steps can go a long way in maintaining healthy, youthful-looking skin.

Chapter 21: Teen Skincare and Acne Management

Provide guidance on teen skincare, focusing on managing acne and promoting healthy habits for lifelong skin health. Teenage years are a transformative period, not just emotionally and mentally, but physically as well. One significant change that happens during this time is with the skin, largely due to the surge of hormones that kick starts sebum (oil) production. This can often lead to acne, which is a common concern among teenagers.

Acne, characterized by the appearance of pimples, blackheads, and whiteheads, is the result of pores getting clogged by oil, dead skin cells, and sometimes bacteria. Understanding the nature of acne is the first step in managing it. It's important to know that it's a normal part of adolescence, and while it can be frustrating, it's entirely manageable with the right approach.

A proper skincare routine is crucial during teenage years, and simplicity is key. Overcomplicating the regimen with too many products can often exacerbate skin issues. The routine should ideally consist of three fundamental steps: cleansing, treating, and moisturizing.

Cleansing twice a day with a gentle, oil-free cleanser can help to remove excess sebum and impurities, preventing pore clogging. Resist the temptation to scrub or over-cleanse the face, as this can strip the skin of its natural oils and trigger even more oil production.

Post-cleansing, treating the skin is the next step. Topical treatments containing benzoyl peroxide or salicylic acid can be beneficial for mild to moderate acne. Benzoyl peroxide works by killing the bacteria that cause acne, while salicylic acid helps unclog the pores. These active ingredients are often found in over-the-counter creams, gels, and lotions.

Moisturizing is a step that can often be overlooked by teenagers, especially those with oily or acne-prone skin, out of fear that it might make the skin even oilier. However, it's crucial to understand that moisturizing helps maintain the skin's natural moisture barrier, protecting it from external irritants and preventing it from overproducing oil. Look for non-comedogenic, oil-free moisturizers that hydrate without clogging pores.

In addition to this, sun protection is essential. Even if it doesn't seem directly related to acne management, protecting the skin from harmful UV rays can prevent damage that may exacerbate existing acne and cause other long-term skin issues. Regular application of a non-comedogenic, broad-spectrum sunscreen with an SPF of at least 30 is recommended.

Diet also plays a role in skin health. While research is still ongoing, some studies suggest a link between diet and acne. Foods high in sugar and dairy products have been implicated in some cases. Maintaining a balanced diet rich in fruits, vegetables, lean proteins, and whole grains can contribute to overall health, including that of the skin.

Lastly, patience is crucial. Acne treatments can take several weeks to show results. Sticking to a consistent routine, even when immediate improvements aren't visible, is critical. For persistent or severe acne, a dermatologist should be consulted. They can prescribe stronger treatments, like retinoids or oral medications, and provide personalized advice based on the individual's specific skin condition.

Teenage skincare is about balance and consistency, and acne management is no different. It's about maintaining a simple but effective routine, making lifestyle choices that support skin health, and seeking professional help when necessary. The goal is not perfection but understanding and taking care of the skin in the best possible way during this dynamic period of life.

Explore the causes of excess oil production and develop strategies for managing oily skin and preventing breakouts. Oily skin is characterized by an excess production of sebum, the skin's natural oil. This overproduction can lead to a shiny complexion, enlarged pores, and mild breakouts. These breakouts can range from occasional pimples, whiteheads, and blackheads, all of which fall into the category of Grade 1 and 2 acne. This is fundamentally different from Grades 3 and 4 acne, which are considered severe forms of the condition and often involve large, painful nodules or cysts.

Understanding your skin and recognizing that oiliness and occasional breakouts are common, especially in certain life stages or during periods of stress, is the first step in managing this skin type. It's also crucial to note that despite its challenges, oily skin has its advantages, including natural moisture and slower aging due to the protective layer of sebum.

The key to managing oily skin and mild breakouts lies in balance. It might seem counterintuitive, but over-cleansing the skin or using harsh, drying products can actually exacerbate oiliness. This is because when the skin is stripped of its natural oils, it can trigger a rebound effect where the skin overproduces oil to compensate.

Cleansing should be done twice a day with a gentle, sulfate-free cleanser. For those who wear makeup or sunscreen, a double cleanse in the evening could be beneficial. This method, which involves using an oil-based cleanser to break down makeup and sunscreen followed by a water-based cleanser, can ensure the skin is thoroughly clean without being stripped of its natural oils.

Exfoliation can also help manage oiliness and prevent breakouts. Regular exfoliation, ideally 1-2 times a week, can help remove dead skin cells that can clog pores and contribute to breakouts. Chemical exfoliants, such as those containing alpha or beta hydroxy acids, are generally preferred over physical exfoliants, as they're less likely to cause skin irritation or damage.

Despite the oily nature of the skin, moisturizing remains an important step. Opt for lightweight, oil-free moisturizers or lotions that hydrate the skin without adding excess oil. Products with hyaluronic acid can be beneficial, as they provide hydration by drawing water into the skin rather than adding oil.

Managing oily skin also involves paying attention to the types of makeup and sunscreens used. Look for products labeled "non-comedogenic," meaning they won't clog pores, and "oil-free" to avoid adding extra oil to the skin. Sunscreen is still a must for all skin types, including oily skin, so look for lightweight, broad-spectrum sunscreens that won't exacerbate oiliness.

On the other hand, Grades 3 and 4 acne involve more severe and persistent breakouts that often cover larger areas of the face or body and can lead to scarring or dark spots. This type of acne typically requires more intensive treatment, which might include prescription medications or professional treatments from a dermatologist. It's crucial to consult with a dermatologist or skin care professional if you suspect you have Grade 3 or 4 acne.

Primarily, managing oily skin and mild breakouts involves a gentle but consistent skincare routine, using appropriate products, and understanding your skin's needs. Remember, everyone's skin is unique, so what works for one person might not work for another. It's always a good idea to seek advice from a skincare professional if you have concerns about your skin or if your skin issues are causing you distress.

Chapter 23: Managing Hormonal Acne and Imbalances

Hormonal acne is a common skin condition that occurs due to fluctuations in the body's hormones. These fluctuations often occur during puberty, but hormonal acne can also affect adults — particularly women during their menstrual cycle, pregnancy, or menopause.

Hormones like testosterone stimulate the sebaceous glands to produce more sebum, an oily substance that helps protect the skin. When the body produces an excess amount of sebum and dead skin cells, the two can build up in the hair follicles and form a soft plug, creating an environment where bacteria can thrive. If the clogged pore becomes infected with bacteria, inflammation results, leading to the well-known red, swollen bumps associated with acne.

Hormonal acne typically appears in the lower part of the face, including the bottom of the cheeks and around the jawline. They're often large, tender, and filled with pus. Factors such as stress and dietary habits can also trigger or worsen hormonal acne.

In terms of managing hormonal acne, there's no one-size-fits-all solution. However, some treatments have been found to be effective. Topical treatments, including retinoids and antibiotics, can help to reduce inflammation and control the acne. Retinoids work by promoting cell turnover and preventing hair follicle plugging, while antibiotics can help kill the excess bacteria on the skin.

For women, hormonal therapies like birth control pills or spironolactone can be beneficial. Birth control pills can help regulate hormonal fluctuations, reducing the severity of acne. Spironolactone, an androgen blocker, can also help in cases where the acne is due to an excess of androgen hormones.

While these treatments can be effective, it's essential to take a holistic approach to managing hormonal acne. This includes maintaining a balanced diet, staying hydrated, and getting regular exercise. Some people find that certain foods — such as dairy, high-glycemic foods, or foods rich in omega-6 fats — can exacerbate their acne, so keeping a food diary can be helpful in identifying potential triggers.

Stress management is another crucial aspect of managing hormonal acne, as stress can influence hormone levels. Techniques such as mindfulness, meditation, yoga, or other stress-relieving activities can be beneficial.

Hormonal imbalances can contribute to various health issues, including acne. Therefore, it can be worthwhile to seek medical advice if you suspect a hormonal imbalance may be contributing to your skin issues. A healthcare professional can provide tests to check hormone levels and suggest appropriate treatment strategies.

While dealing with hormonal acne can be frustrating, it's important to remember that everyone's skin is different. What works for one person might not work for another, and finding the right treatment can take time. The journey to clear skin often involves a combination of treatments, lifestyle changes, and a lot of patience. With perseverance and the right support, hormonal acne can be managed effectively.

Chapter 24: Skincare for Mature Skin

Cater to the specific needs of mature skin, discussing treatments for age-related concerns and promoting a youthful complexion. Mature skin care is all about embracing the natural aging process while caring for the skin to maintain its health and vitality. As the skin ages, it undergoes several changes: it tends to become thinner, lose elasticity, and produce less oil and collagen. These changes can result in dryness, fine lines, wrinkles, and sagging. But, with a well-thought-out skincare routine and lifestyle adjustments, it's possible to manage these changes effectively.

Cleansing is the foundational step of any skincare routine, irrespective of age. However, for mature skin, the choice of cleanser is essential. Harsh, soap-based cleansers can strip the skin of its natural oils, leading to dryness and irritation. Instead, opt for gentle, hydrating cleansers that remove impurities without compromising the skin's moisture barrier.

Exfoliation becomes increasingly important with age, as the skin's natural cell turnover slows down. Regular, gentle exfoliation can help remove dead skin cells and stimulate the renewal process, revealing brighter, smoother skin. Chemical exfoliants, like alpha hydroxy acids (AHAs), can be particularly beneficial for mature skin, as they can also help improve skin texture and reduce the appearance of age spots.

As we age, the skin naturally produces less collagen, a protein responsible for the skin's strength and elasticity. Stimulating collagen production is therefore a key goal in mature skincare. Topical vitamin A derivatives, known as retinoids, are one of the most studied and proven ingredients to boost collagen production, reduce the appearance of wrinkles, and improve skin texture. Retinoids should be introduced gradually into the skincare routine, starting with lower concentrations, to minimize potential irritation.

In addition to retinoids, peptides and vitamin C are other potent ingredients that can help stimulate collagen production. Peptides are small proteins that can penetrate the skin and signal it to produce more collagen. Vitamin C is a potent antioxidant that not only helps protect the skin from environmental damage but also boosts collagen production and brightens the skin.

Hydration is another critical aspect of mature skincare. As oil production decreases with age, the skin can become dry and more susceptible to damage. Incorporating a deeply hydrating moisturizer, or even a hyaluronic acid serum, can help replenish the skin's moisture and improve its texture and firmness.

Sun protection remains critical at any age. Daily use of a broad-spectrum sunscreen can prevent further damage and premature aging caused by harmful UV rays. When it comes to mature skin, prevention is just as important as repair.

Lastly, lifestyle factors play a significant role in skin health. Consuming a balanced diet rich in antioxidants, lean proteins, and healthy fats can nourish the skin from the inside out and support overall skin health. Regular exercise can also promote healthy circulation and contribute to a youthful glow.

In essence, mature skincare is about nurturing the skin with effective, targeted products and maintaining a healthy lifestyle. It's about embracing the aging process while giving the skin what it needs to age gracefully. Despite the inevitable changes that come with age, with the right care and attention, mature skin can remain healthy, vibrant, and beautiful for many years.

Chapter 25: Preventative Skincare in Your 20s and 30s

Guide clients in their 20s and 30s on the importance of preventative skincare and establishing healthy habits. The journey of preventative skincare often starts in your 20s and 30s. This period is a critical time to develop good skincare habits that will help maintain healthy, youthful skin in the years to come. During this stage, the skin still has robust collagen and elastin production, but early signs of aging, such as fine lines and sunspots, can start to appear, especially if preventive measures aren't taken.

In your 20s, the focus should be on maintaining the skin's health and preventing damage. An essential first step in any skincare routine is cleansing. Regular and thorough cleansing helps to keep the pores clear of excess sebum and dirt, preventing breakouts and providing a clean slate for the absorption of other skincare products. It's crucial to use a gentle, pH-balanced cleanser to avoid stripping the skin of its natural oils.

Exfoliation is another critical component of skincare in your 20s. This process helps remove dead skin cells, promotes skin renewal, and helps maintain a clear, radiant complexion. However, it's essential to not overdo it, as excessive exfoliation can strip the skin's protective barrier. Depending on the skin's sensitivity, 1-2 times per week is usually sufficient.

Next, hydration is key. While your skin may still produce plenty of natural oils in your 20s, external factors like air conditioning, heating, and pollution can strip the skin of moisture, leading to dryness or dehydration. A good quality moisturizer suited to your skin type will help seal in moisture and keep the skin supple and hydrated.

Sunscreen is a non-negotiable part of preventative skincare. Daily application of a broad-spectrum sunscreen with an SPF of at least 30 can protect the skin from harmful UV rays and prevent premature aging. Remember, the sun is the number one cause of skin aging, so never skip this step!

Incorporating antioxidants into your skincare routine is also a smart move in your 20s. Antioxidants like vitamin C can neutralize harmful free radicals that can damage the skin cells and accelerate aging. A topical vitamin C serum can brighten the skin, boost collagen production, and strengthen the skin's defense against environmental damage.

As you transition into your 30s, your skincare routine should evolve to address the slowing down of skin cell turnover and the gradual decrease in collagen production. This is the perfect time to introduce retinoids into your skincare routine. Derived from vitamin A, retinoids can help accelerate cell turnover, improve skin texture, and stimulate collagen production.

Hydration becomes even more important in your 30s, as the skin's natural ability to retain moisture starts to decrease. Incorporating hydrating serums or creams with hyaluronic acid can help keep the skin plump and hydrated. Hyaluronic acid can hold up to 1000 times its weight in water, making it a superstar ingredient for hydration.

Lastly, don't forget about the skin on your neck and chest. These areas are often overlooked but are just as exposed to the elements as your face. The skin here is thinner and has fewer oil glands, which makes it more susceptible to premature aging. Be sure to extend all aspects of your skincare routine to these areas too.

Preventative skincare in your 20s and 30s is about maintaining the health of your skin, preventing premature aging, and laying a strong foundation for the future of your skin. It's about developing and maintaining good skincare habits, and understanding that prevention is easier than correction when it comes to skin aging.

Chapter 26: Understanding Skin Conditions: Psoriasis and Eczema

Let's delve into the complexities of psoriasis and eczema, understanding their triggers and providing specialized treatments. Psoriasis and eczema are common skin conditions that can cause discomfort and self-consciousness, but they are distinctly different conditions, each with unique causes, symptoms, and treatments.

Psoriasis is a chronic autoimmune condition that speeds up the life cycle of skin cells. This accelerated turnover results in the build-up of cells on the surface of the skin, leading to patches of red, inflamed skin covered with silvery scales. These patches can be itchy or sore, and are most often found on the elbows, knees, scalp, back, face, palms, and feet. The exact cause of psoriasis isn't fully understood, but it's believed to be related to an overactive immune system and has a strong genetic component. Psoriasis is not contagious and can occur at any age, although it's most commonly diagnosed in adults.

There are several types of psoriasis, each with distinct characteristics. Plaque psoriasis, the most common type, causes raised, inflamed, red skin covered with silvery, white scales. Other types include guttate psoriasis, which often starts in childhood and causes small, dot-like lesions, and pustular psoriasis, which is characterized by blisters of non-infectious pus.

The treatment for psoriasis aims to slow skin cell turnover and reduce inflammation, itchiness, and the appearance of scales. This might involve topical treatments, oral or injected medications, or light therapy. Many people with psoriasis also benefit from lifestyle changes, such as maintaining a healthy weight, avoiding tobacco and alcohol, and managing stress.

Eczema, also known as atopic dermatitis, is a chronic condition that makes the skin red, itchy, and inflamed. It's common in children but can occur at any age. Eczema is long-lasting and tends to flare periodically. It may be accompanied by asthma or hay fever. No cure exists for eczema, but treatments and self-care measures can relieve itching and prevent new outbreaks.

The exact cause of eczema is unknown, but it's believed to involve a combination of genetic, environmental, and immune system factors. Eczema is not contagious, and while its symptoms can be similar to psoriasis — red, inflamed, itchy skin — eczema tends to occur in different areas of the body, such as the insides of the elbows or knees, and the skin often looks dark, leathery, or scaly.

Eczema treatment focuses on healing the skin and preventing flare-ups. This can involve the use of moisturizers to hydrate the skin, topical medications to reduce inflammation and itching, and lifestyle changes to avoid triggers. For some people, triggers might include certain soaps or detergents, dust mites, stress, or certain foods.

Both psoriasis and eczema can have a significant impact on quality of life, leading to discomfort, sleep disturbance, and feelings of self-consciousness. However, with appropriate treatment and management, the symptoms of both conditions can be effectively controlled. It's always important to consult with a healthcare professional, such as a dermatologist, for a proper diagnosis and treatment plan.

Chapter 27: Seasonal Skincare Adjustments

Understand how environmental factors affect the skin and recommend seasonal adjustments to skincare routines. Seasonal changes can have a significant impact on your skin's health and appearance. As the weather shifts, so too do the needs of your skin. Being attuned to these changes and adjusting your skincare routine accordingly can help keep your skin balanced, comfortable, and looking its best all year round.

In the warmer months of spring and summer, higher temperatures and increased humidity can make your skin produce more oil, leading to a shinier complexion and potentially more breakouts. It's a good time to switch to lighter, gel-based cleansers and moisturizers that cleanse and hydrate without adding extra oil to your skin. Sun protection becomes even more crucial during these months due to the longer daylight hours and more potent UV rays. Wearing a broad-spectrum sunscreen with an SPF of 30 or higher, reapplying it every two hours, and wearing protective clothing and accessories can help prevent sun damage.

In contrast, the cooler, drier air of autumn and winter can leave your skin feeling dry, tight, and flaky. During these months, it's beneficial to incorporate more hydrating and moisturizing products into your routine. Creamy, lipid-rich cleansers can help to preserve the skin's natural oils, while thicker moisturizers, especially those containing humectants like hyaluronic acid and emollients like shea butter, can help to lock in moisture and form a protective barrier against the harsh elements.

Exfoliation continues to be important throughout the year, but the type of exfoliant you use may change with the seasons. In the warmer months, a light exfoliant may be sufficient to keep your skin glowing. However, in the colder months, a more intensive exfoliant may be required to remove the buildup of dry, dead skin cells. However, always remember to exfoliate gently and not too frequently to avoid damaging the skin's barrier.

No matter the season, there are a few constants in any good skincare routine. These include cleansing twice a day to remove dirt, oil, and makeup, applying a good quality moisturizer to hydrate and protect your skin, and using sunscreen daily to guard against UV damage. Remember, while the sun may not feel as strong in the cooler months, UV rays are still present and can still cause damage.

Different seasons bring different challenges, and your skin's needs can vary widely throughout the year. It's essential to listen to your skin and make adjustments as needed. Don't be afraid to experiment with different products and routines until you find what works best for your skin in each season. After all, great skincare is not a one-size-fits-all solution but a personalized routine that evolves with you and your skin's needs.

Don't overlook the impact of your lifestyle on your skin, either. Keeping a balanced diet, drinking plenty of water, getting enough sleep, and managing stress can support your skin health throughout the year. Despite the changing weather, with the right care and attention, you can maintain healthy, glowing skin no matter the season.

Chapter 28: Special Occasion Skincare

Provide tips and treatments to help clients achieve glowing skin for special events. Prepping your skin for a special occasion requires a thoughtful and effective skincare strategy. Whether you're getting ready for a wedding, a milestone birthday, or any other big event, you'll want your skin to look its best. While your daily skincare routine plays a significant role in maintaining your skin health, professional treatments can provide a boost to enhance your skin's glow and address specific concerns.

Professional facial treatments are a popular choice for special occasion prep. A thorough, deep-cleansing facial can provide an immediate radiance to your skin. It usually involves steps like cleansing, exfoliating, extracting, massaging, and applying a mask, all tailored to your skin type and concerns. These facials can unclog your pores, remove dull skin cells, boost circulation, and hydrate your skin, leaving you with a clear, glowing complexion.

If you're looking to address specific skin issues, such as fine lines, hyperpigmentation, or acne scars, you might consider treatments like chemical peels or microdermabrasion. Chemical peels involve the application of a chemical solution to your skin, which causes it to exfoliate and eventually peel off, revealing smoother, less wrinkled skin underneath. Microdermabrasion, on the other hand, is a minimally invasive procedure that uses a special applicator to gently sand away the thick outer layer of the skin, rejuvenating your skin's appearance.

For a significant boost in skin's hydration and plumpness, consider a hyaluronic acid filler or a treatment like the HydraFacial. Hyaluronic acid fillers can add volume, smooth wrinkles, and give an overall plumped, youthful look. The HydraFacial is a multi-step treatment that cleanses, exfoliates, extracts, and hydrates the skin, while also infusing it with a blend of beneficial ingredients like antioxidants and peptides.

If you're seeking firmer, tighter skin, consider treatments like microcurrent or radiofrequency. Microcurrent is a low-level current that mimics the body's natural current, resulting in improved facial contour and skin tone. Radiofrequency treatments, on the other hand, use energy to heat the skin, stimulating collagen and elastin production for firmer, smoother skin.

Laser treatments are another popular choice for special occasion skincare prep. Different types of laser treatments can target various skin concerns, from wrinkles to sun damage to acne scars. For example, fractionated laser treatments create micro-injuries in the skin to stimulate the skin's healing response and boost collagen production.

It's crucial to plan these treatments well in advance of your special occasion. Some treatments, like peels and lasers, can leave your skin looking worse before it gets better. You'll also want to allow your skin time to recover and reach its peak post-treatment glow.

Additionally, it's important to remember that while these professional treatments can provide remarkable results, they're not a replacement for a consistent, effective daily skincare routine. In the lead-up to your special event, be diligent about your skincare basics: cleansing, moisturizing, and protecting your skin from the sun.

Professional skincare treatments offer a way to address specific concerns and give your skin a significant boost. But ultimately, the best foundation for glowing skin on your special day is a well-cared-for complexion. By combining regular skincare with strategic professional treatments, you can ensure your skin looks its best, no matter the occasion.

Learn to identify common skincare allergens and how to cater to clients with sensitive skin. When it comes to skincare, understanding allergies and sensitivities is crucial. Our skin acts as the first line of defense against external irritants, but it can also react negatively to certain substances, resulting in allergic reactions or sensitivities. Distinguishing between these two conditions is key as it affects both treatment and prevention.

An allergic reaction in skin care typically occurs when the immune system overreacts to a particular substance, or allergen, that it considers harmful, even though it might be harmless to most people. This reaction is systemic, which means it involves the whole body. Common signs of an allergic reaction include hives, itching, redness, and swelling. In some cases, a severe allergic reaction, or anaphylaxis, can occur, leading to difficulty breathing and a drop in blood pressure.

In skincare, common allergens include ingredients like fragrances and preservatives, which are found in many skincare products. Nickel, which can be found in cosmetic tools, is another common allergen. Patch testing is a common method used by dermatologists to identify specific allergens. During a patch test, small amounts of potential allergens are applied to the skin via adhesive patches, which are usually worn for a few days to observe for reactions.

On the other hand, a sensitivity, or irritation, is a more localized response that occurs when the skin becomes inflamed due to certain triggers. It typically occurs at the site of contact and doesn't involve the immune system. Symptoms of skin sensitivity can include redness, itching, burning, and stinging.

In skincare, sensitive skin can react negatively to a wide range of triggers, including harsh cleansers, certain active ingredients like retinol or alpha hydroxy acids, physical exfoliants, and even environmental factors like wind and extreme temperatures. Individuals with sensitive skin should aim for gentle, hypoallergenic products and be mindful of introducing new products one at a time to monitor for potential reactions.

Interestingly, skin sensitivities can also develop over time due to factors like overuse of harsh skincare products, which can strip the skin's protective barrier and make it more vulnerable to irritants. Thus, if you notice your skin becoming increasingly reactive, it might be time to evaluate your skincare routine and consult with a dermatologist or a certified esthetician.

Managing skin allergies and sensitivities often requires a two-pronged approach: avoidance of known triggers and strengthening of the skin barrier. If you have identified specific allergens or irritants, it's important to check the ingredient lists of skincare products to ensure they're not present. Furthermore, maintaining a healthy skin barrier with a gentle skincare routine can help protect your skin from potential irritants and allergens.

Ultimately, understanding skin allergies and sensitivities is crucial to achieving healthy skin. It helps us make informed decisions about the products we use, the routines we follow, and when to seek professional advice. By being proactive and mindful, we can better navigate the vast world of skincare and find what truly works for our individual needs.

Chapter 30: Skincare for People of Color

Address specific skincare concerns and treatments for individuals with deeper skin tones. Skincare is deeply personal and heavily influenced by individual skin characteristics, which can often be related to our ethnic backgrounds. People of different ethnicities can have unique skin issues that need specific care. For Hispanic, African American, and people of color, understanding their skin's unique needs can help formulate the best skincare regimen.

For Hispanic individuals, one common skin issue is hyperpigmentation or dark spots. This condition can be a result of sun damage, acne, hormonal changes, or even injuries to the skin. Hyperpigmentation can often be more noticeable on Hispanic skin due to the higher amount of melanin. Sun protection is crucial in preventing and managing hyperpigmentation, and using a broad-spectrum sunscreen with an SPF of at least 30 is recommended. Other helpful treatments include topical retinoids, vitamin C, and products with ingredients like hydroquinone or niacinamide that can lighten dark spots.

In addition, Hispanic skin can be more prone to oiliness and acne due to higher sebum production. Using a gentle cleanser that can effectively remove oil and dirt without stripping the skin's natural moisture is key. Incorporating ingredients like salicylic acid or benzoyl peroxide, which can help unclog pores and reduce acne, can also be beneficial.

When it comes to African American skin, post-inflammatory hyperpigmentation (PIH) is a common concern. PIH occurs when an area of the skin becomes darker following an injury or inflammation, such as acne. It can be more prevalent and last longer in African American skin due to the increased melanin. Treatment options are similar to those for hyperpigmentation in Hispanic skin, with sun protection playing an essential role in prevention and management.

African American skin can also be more prone to certain conditions like keloids, which are raised scars that extend beyond the original injury. Early treatment is important to manage keloids, and options include silicone sheets, corticosteroid injections, and laser treatments.

For people of color in general, it's important to remember that while their skin may be more resilient to sun damage due to higher melanin levels, sun protection is still necessary. Damage from UV radiation can still lead to premature aging and increase the risk of skin cancer. A broad-spectrum sunscreen is crucial for all skin types and colors.

Furthermore, finding the right skincare products can sometimes be challenging for people of color, as certain products can leave a white or gray cast on the skin. Look for sunscreens labeled as 'sheer' or 'invisible', and opt for tinted products if necessary.

Everyone's skin is unique, and understanding your skin's specific needs can help you care for it effectively. For Hispanic, African American, and people of color, this understanding is just as important. With the right knowledge and the right products, maintaining healthy, glowing skin is achievable for everyone, regardless of their skin color or ethnicity.

Chapter 31: The Benefits of Facial Steaming

Explore the benefits of facial steaming and how it enhances the effectiveness of skincare products. Facial steaming, a popular skincare practice, has been touted for its numerous benefits. The warmth of the steam causes the skin to heat up, which promotes sweating and the opening of pores. This process can aid in the removal of dirt, bacteria, and dead skin cells that are often trapped in the pores, thus reducing the occurrence of breakouts and pimples. Steaming can also help increase circulation, bringing more oxygen and nutrients to the skin, resulting in a naturally healthy and radiant glow.

Another key benefit of facial steaming is that it can enhance the effectiveness of your skincare products. By opening the pores, steam allows skincare products to penetrate deeper into the skin, making them more effective. This can be particularly beneficial when you're using products with active ingredients, such as serums or treatment masks, as it helps these products deliver their benefits more efficiently.

Facial steaming also has the advantage of being a natural and inexpensive skincare method. All you really need is hot water and a bowl or a dedicated facial steamer. Some people like to add herbs, essential oils, or tea to their steaming water for added therapeutic benefits. For instance, adding chamomile can provide a soothing effect, while adding peppermint can stimulate and refresh the skin.

However, while facial steaming can offer these benefits, it's not without its potential downsides. For those with sensitive skin or certain skin conditions, such as rosacea, facial steaming can actually exacerbate their issues. The heat from the steam can cause redness and irritation, leading to more pronounced symptoms.

Another risk of facial steaming is burns. If the steam is too hot or if you're too close to the source, it can lead to burns, which can be harmful to the skin and cause scarring. Therefore, it's important to test the temperature of the steam with your hand first and to keep a safe distance.

Furthermore, while steam can open the pores and help remove impurities, it doesn't discriminate between the bad oil (sebum) and the good oil (lipids) in your skin. If you steam your face too often or for too long, you risk stripping your skin of its natural oils, leading to dryness and potential disruption of your skin's natural barrier.

As with any skincare practice, it's important to consider your individual skin needs and conditions when deciding whether to incorporate facial steaming into your routine. For some, it can be a beneficial addition that boosts the effectiveness of their skincare products and imparts a healthy glow. For others, especially those with sensitive skin or skin conditions, it's important to exercise caution. When used wisely and appropriately, facial steaming can be a pleasant and beneficial part of a skincare routine.

Chapter 32: Aromatherapy and Essential Oils in Skincare

Discover the therapeutic benefits of essential oils in skincare and how they complement various treatments. Aromatherapy and the use of essential oils have been practiced for centuries, offering a range of benefits for both physical and emotional health. These potent oils, derived from plants, carry the essence of the plants' beneficial properties, offering an array of therapeutic benefits that can be utilized in skincare.

Incorporating essential oils into skincare can provide a myriad of benefits. Lavender, for instance, is known for its soothing properties and can aid in calming irritated skin while providing a relaxing scent. Tea tree oil has powerful antimicrobial properties, making it a popular choice for combating acne. Chamomile oil is recognized for its anti-inflammatory qualities that can help calm skin redness and irritation.

Essential oils are also used for their therapeutic aroma. When inhaled, these fragrances can stimulate areas of your limbic system, which is a part of your brain that plays a role in emotions, behaviors, sense of smell, and long-term memory. As a result, incorporating aromatherapy into your skincare routine can not only benefit your skin but also enhance your overall well-being.

Despite their benefits, essential oils should be used with caution. They are highly concentrated and, if not properly diluted, can cause skin irritation or allergic reactions. Patch testing is crucial before applying any essential oil to your skin. This involves applying a small amount of the diluted essential oil to a patch of skin and monitoring for any reactions over 24 hours.

Allergic reactions to essential oils can occur and often manifest as contact dermatitis - a red, itchy rash that occurs where the oil touches the skin. In some cases, it can cause more severe reactions, like hives or blisters. Common culprits include oils from the citrus family, like lemon or bergamot, as well as cinnamon, jasmine, and ylang-ylang.

Not all essential oils are suitable for all skin types. For instance, while tea tree oil might be excellent for oily and acne-prone skin, it might be too drying for individuals with dry or sensitive skin. Similarly, certain essential oils, like bergamot and other citrus oils, can cause photosensitivity, making your skin more susceptible to sun damage.

It's also worth noting that the quality of essential oils can vary widely. Pure, high-quality oils are more likely to provide the therapeutic benefits you're looking for and less likely to cause irritation or adverse reactions. Look for oils that are labeled as "100% pure" and avoid oils with additives or synthetic fragrances.

In the end, when used properly, aromatherapy and essential oils can be a beneficial addition to your skincare regimen. They can offer unique benefits and transform your skincare routine into a more sensory and holistic experience. However, it's crucial to educate yourself about their proper use and potential risks to ensure you're utilizing them in a safe and beneficial manner.

Chapter 33: Dealing with Redness and Irritation

Discuss the causes of redness and irritation and explore soothing treatments for sensitive skin. Redness and irritation on the face can be caused by various factors including sensitive skin, allergic reactions, sunburn, wind exposure, rosacea, and certain skin conditions such as dermatitis. Understanding the cause of your skin redness and irritation is crucial to finding the most effective way to deal with it.

To alleviate redness and irritation, it's often helpful to start with gentle, soothing skincare products. These should be free from irritants such as alcohol, fragrances, and harsh chemicals. Ingredients like aloe vera, chamomile, cucumber, and green tea can have calming effects on the skin. Aloe vera, for instance, is well-known for its soothing and anti-inflammatory properties, making it an excellent ingredient for calming red and irritated skin.

If the redness and irritation are caused by dryness, moisturizing the skin can help. Hydrating ingredients such as hyaluronic acid and glycerin can restore moisture to the skin, reducing dryness and subsequent irritation. Hyaluronic acid is especially beneficial as it can hold up to 1000 times its weight in water, helping to keep your skin hydrated and plump.

It's also crucial to protect irritated skin from sun exposure, which can further exacerbate redness and irritation. Using a broad-spectrum sunscreen with an SPF of at least 30 can shield your skin from damaging UV rays. Mineral sunscreens, containing ingredients like zinc oxide and titanium dioxide, are often less irritating for sensitive skin compared to chemical sunscreens.

For persistent redness and irritation, over-the-counter creams containing mild corticosteroids can help. These creams can reduce inflammation and soothe the skin. However, these should be used sparingly and under a healthcare provider's guidance as long-term use can lead to skin thinning.

Cold compresses or face masks can also provide immediate relief for irritated skin. The coolness can constrict blood vessels, reducing redness, and offer a soothing sensation. Look for masks with soothing ingredients, like the ones mentioned above, for an added boost of relief.

Skin redness and irritation can also be an indicator of underlying skin conditions like rosacea or dermatitis. If you find that your redness and irritation persist despite your best efforts, or if it is accompanied by other symptoms like itching, burning, or swelling, it may be time to seek professional help. A dermatologist can evaluate your skin, provide a proper diagnosis, and recommend appropriate treatments. Remember, each person's skin is unique, and what works for one person may not work for another. Therefore, it's important to listen to your skin, recognize its needs, and adapt your skincare routine accordingly.

Chapter 34: Skincare in Different Climates

The climate you live in can significantly influence your skincare routine. From the humidity levels of a tropical climate to the dry, cold air of winter months, each environment presents its own set of challenges and considerations for skin health.

In hot, humid climates, the high levels of moisture in the air can make your skin feel greasier. This can lead to clogged pores and an increase in acne breakouts. It's important to keep the skin clean and free from excess oil in these conditions. Light, non-comedogenic products that won't clog pores are often preferred. Ingredients like niacinamide and salicylic acid can help regulate sebum production and prevent breakouts. Sun protection is also crucial in hot climates, as prolonged sun exposure can lead to sunburn, premature aging, and an increased risk of skin cancer.

In contrast, dry, arid climates can strip your skin of its natural oils, leading to dryness and dehydration. To counteract this, it's important to focus on hydration and maintaining the skin's moisture barrier. Products with hyaluronic acid, a potent humectant that can hold a large amount of water, are ideal for these conditions. Emollients like ceramides and squalene can also help restore the skin's lipid barrier, preventing moisture loss.

Cold, winter climates pose another set of challenges. The low temperatures and low humidity levels can leave skin feeling dry, tight, and irritated. In such conditions, it's beneficial to use rich, nourishing creams that can protect the skin from the harsh environment. Ingredients like shea butter, glycerin, and ceramides can provide the skin with necessary hydration and help repair the skin's natural barrier function. Don't forget about sun protection, as UV rays can still cause damage even in the cold months.

Lastly, for those in temperate climates where there are distinct seasonal changes, it's often necessary to adjust your skincare routine as the seasons change. During the warmer months, lighter, oil-controlling products might be preferred. As it transitions to colder months, a shift towards more moisturizing, protective skincare products can help keep the skin healthy and hydrated.

While these guidelines provide a starting point, it's crucial to remember that everyone's skin is unique. Listening to your skin and observing how it reacts to different climates can provide valuable insights. By tailoring your skincare routine to both your individual skin needs and the specific demands of your climate, you can help ensure your skin stays healthy and vibrant in any weather.

Chapter 35: Professionally Incorporating Technology in Skincare

Explore technological advancements like LED therapy, microcurrent, and radiofrequency for advanced skincare treatments. The advent of technology has transformed the skincare industry, adding a high-tech twist to traditional skincare routines. From skincare devices that cleanse, tone, and stimulate the skin, to advanced tools that help with anti-aging, there's a plethora of technology available to enhance your skincare regimen.

Devices such as cleansing brushes, microcurrent devices, and sonic cleansers have gained popularity due to their ability to deep clean the skin, dislodge impurities from pores, and increase circulation. For example, cleansing brushes can provide a deep clean that manual cleansing may not offer, and microcurrent devices use low-level electrical currents to stimulate facial muscles, promoting collagen and elastin production for a tighter, more youthful appearance.

Light therapy devices are another popular category of skincare technology. These devices, which use specific wavelengths of light, can target various skin issues. Blue light therapy is often used to combat acne, as it can kill acne-causing bacteria. Red light therapy, on the other hand, can stimulate collagen production and help reduce signs of aging.

Microdermabrasion devices offer a way to exfoliate the skin at home. These devices use tiny crystals or a diamond tip to remove the top layer of dead skin cells, helping to brighten the complexion and promote the absorption of skincare products.

Then there are skin analysis tools that use artificial intelligence and high-resolution imaging to assess the skin's condition, including identifying signs of aging, sun damage, dehydration, and more. These tools can provide personalized skincare recommendations based on the analysis, allowing for a truly customized skincare routine.

In the professional setting, dermatologists and estheticians utilize advanced technologies such as laser treatments, radiofrequency, and intense pulsed light (IPL) for a range of skin concerns, from hair removal and pigmentation to anti-aging and skin tightening. These technologies offer targeted and often more potent solutions for skin issues, but should always be administered by a trained professional due to their strength and potential side effects.

While incorporating technology into your skincare routine can be beneficial, it's important to remember that these devices should complement, not replace, a regular skincare routine. Basic skincare steps like cleansing, moisturizing, and sun protection are still vital for maintaining skin health. It's also essential to use these devices as instructed by the manufacturer or a professional to avoid any potential skin damage. Remember, the best skincare routine is the one that suits your individual needs and concerns, whether that includes a skin therapist assisting with high-tech devices or not.

Chapter 36: Benefits of Visiting an Esthetician Often

Visiting an esthetician on a regular basis offers a host of benefits that can greatly contribute to the health and appearance of your skin. Estheticians are skincare professionals trained in various treatments and modalities designed to improve and maintain the skin's health.

One of the key benefits of visiting an esthetician is their ability to provide professional-grade treatments that can't be replicated at home. These might include deep cleansing facials, chemical peels, microdermabrasion, dermaplaning, or extractions, all of which can deeply cleanse, exfoliate, and rejuvenate the skin in ways that over-the-counter products may not be able to.

An esthetician can also offer personalized skincare advice based on an in-depth understanding of your skin type and needs. They are trained to analyze your skin, recognize conditions that you may not be aware of, and recommend appropriate treatments and products. This expert advice can help you better understand your skin and build a more effective skincare routine.

Estheticians also provide a level of relaxation and stress relief that's hard to achieve at home. Many esthetician services, such as facials, incorporate elements of massage and relaxation that can promote overall wellness. This relaxation can lead to decreased stress levels, which not only benefits your overall health but can also have positive effects on your skin.

Regular visits to an esthetician can help keep skin issues at bay. For those prone to acne, blackheads, or other skin concerns, frequent professional treatments can help manage these issues, and potentially prevent them from becoming more serious over time. An esthetician can also monitor your skin's health over time, spotting any changes or potential issues early.

While it might seem like a luxury, seeing an esthetician can be an investment in your skin's long-term health and beauty. The exact frequency of visits will depend on your individual skin needs and goals, but a typical recommendation might be once a month, as this aligns with the skin's natural renewal cycle. Whether you're looking for targeted treatments for specific skin concerns, professional advice, or simply the chance to relax and treat yourself, regular visits to an esthetician can be a valuable part of your skincare routine.

Chapter 37: Esthetician vs. Dermatologist

Estheticians and dermatologists both play crucial roles in skincare, but they serve different purposes and operate in distinct professional domains. Understanding the difference between these two professions can help you decide who to turn to for your specific skin concerns.

Dermatologists are medical doctors who specialize in the health of the skin, hair, and nails. They are trained to diagnose and treat more than 3,000 different conditions, ranging from acne and eczema to skin cancer. Dermatologists complete rigorous medical training, which includes a medical degree, a residency in dermatology, and often further specialized training. They are equipped to handle serious skin diseases, perform surgical procedures, and prescribe medication. If you have a skin condition that needs medical attention, such as severe acne, rosacea, psoriasis, or suspicious moles, a dermatologist is the professional to see.

Estheticians, on the other hand, focus on the cosmetic appearance of the skin. They are licensed professionals who are trained to perform a variety of skin treatments designed to improve, maintain, or rejuvenate the skin. These may include facials, chemical peels, microdermabrasion, waxing, and more. Estheticians can analyze your skin type, recommend suitable skincare products, and provide advice on daily skincare routines. They can also address common skin concerns like fine lines, wrinkles, dryness, or mild acne, and perform treatments that promote relaxation and stress relief.

It's important to note that while estheticians can offer valuable advice and perform beneficial treatments, they are not medical doctors and cannot diagnose skin diseases, prescribe medication, or perform surgical procedures. If you're unsure about a skin issue, it's always advisable to consult a dermatologist.

The choice between an esthetician and a dermatologist depends on your needs. If you're looking for a deep-cleansing facial, advice on skincare products, or treatments for common skin concerns like dullness or mild acne, an esthetician can be a great choice. If you have a serious skin condition, need medical advice, or are considering a surgical procedure, a dermatologist is the right professional to see.

In many cases, people might benefit from seeing both. A dermatologist can provide treatment for serious skin conditions and monitor the overall health of your skin, while regular visits to an esthetician can help maintain the health and appearance of your skin, address minor skin concerns, and offer relaxation and stress relief. By understanding the differences and capabilities of each profession, you can make an informed decision about who to see for your skincare needs.

Chapter 38: Handling Common Client Concerns and Complaints

When clients bring their skin concerns or complaints to estheticians, these skincare professionals use their knowledge and expertise to provide solutions. The process typically starts with a thorough skin analysis, where the esthetician examines the client's skin type, condition, and any specific concerns they might have.

Estheticians often use specialized tools or magnifying lamps during the skin analysis to get a closer look at the skin's surface and identify any underlying issues. This can reveal problems that may not be visible to the naked eye, such as early signs of sun damage or aging, clogged pores, dryness, or uneven skin tone.

An esthetician then listens attentively to the client's concerns, whether it's about a particular skin condition like acne or rosacea, or more general concerns like dullness or signs of aging. This conversation helps the esthetician understand the client's goals and expectations and the specific issues they're facing. Active listening and empathy are key skills for estheticians during this stage, as understanding and acknowledging clients' worries can build trust and facilitate more effective treatment.

After the skin analysis and conversation, an esthetician will tailor a treatment plan that addresses the client's specific concerns. This might involve recommending certain professional treatments, such as facials, chemical peels, or microdermabrasion. The treatment plan often also includes advice on a daily skincare routine, with product recommendations that are suitable for the client's skin type and condition.

During subsequent visits, an esthetician will monitor the client's progress and make any necessary adjustments to the treatment plan. This may involve changing or introducing new treatments or products, or providing additional advice on skincare habits. The goal is always to improve the client's skin health and help them feel confident and comfortable in their skin.

When dealing with client complaints, it's essential for an esthetician to maintain a professional and respectful approach. If a client is unhappy with a treatment or product, the esthetician will seek to understand the issue, provide a clear explanation or solution, and rectify the situation as best as they can. Sometimes, the esthetician may need to refer the client to a dermatologist or another healthcare professional, particularly if the skin concern is beyond their scope of practice.

Ultimately, as an esthetician's role is to guide and assist clients on their skincare journey, providing expertise, support, and care to help clients achieve their skin goals and address their concerns.

Chapter 39: The Rise of Facial Parties with an Esthetician

In recent years, the allure of self-care and bonding experiences has given birth to an exciting trend: facial parties led by professionals. If you've ever attended a party where cosmetics were sold or had a friend invite you to a "spa day" at their home, you might be familiar with the concept. But when you add an esthetician to the mix, the experience goes beyond simple relaxation and enters the realm of expert skincare.

The Magic of Group Facials

Picture this: a serene ambiance filled with the scent of essential oils, soft lighting, and gentle music playing in the background. Your closest friends are gathered, each wearing plush robes and awaiting their turn for a skin consultation. This is a facial party with a licensed esthetician. Instead of the hurried atmosphere of a spa or salon, there's an intimate, relaxed vibe that makes skincare feel more like a bonding ritual than a regimen.

But the magic doesn't stop there. The true value lies in the expert guidance of the esthetician. They offer tailored advice to each participant, analyzing individual skin types, discussing concerns, and even demonstrating the correct techniques to apply products. You're not just indulging in a facial; you're participating in an interactive skincare masterclass.

Benefits and Considerations

For those attending, the benefits are manifold. Firstly, there's the educational aspect. It's one thing to watch a skincare tutorial online, but having a professional analyze your specific skin needs and teach you in person is invaluable. Secondly, it fosters community. Sharing beauty secrets, discussing skin woes, and laughing over clay-masked selfies can be a delightful way to connect.

However, there are considerations to keep in mind. Sanitation is paramount. It's crucial to ensure that the esthetician adheres to strict hygiene practices to prevent the spread of bacteria or potential irritations. Also, while group settings can be fun, they might not always provide the depth of personalization that a one-on-one session can offer.

The Future of Facial Parties

As people continue to prioritize self-care and seek out novel experiences, the trend of facial parties with estheticians is likely to grow. It blends the appeal of personal pampering with the joy of social connection. For many, it's not just about achieving radiant skin; it's about deepening bonds, creating memories, and fostering a sense of community around the shared goal of self-improvement.

So, the next time you're thinking of a unique way to celebrate a birthday, a bridal shower, or just a much-needed girls' night in, consider hiring an esthetician and elevating your gathering to a transformative skincare experience. Who knows, you might just find your skin's glow matches the warmth of the memories you create.

Chapter 40: Embracing Who You Are

Embracing your skin as it is, in all its uniqueness and imperfection, is a fundamental aspect of self-love and acceptance. This can be a transformative experience, fostering a more positive self-image and boosting overall confidence. It's important to remember that no one has perfect skin — everyone experiences issues like breakouts, blemishes, or dryness from time to time. Understanding and accepting this can help reduce the pressure to achieve an unrealistic standard of 'perfect' skin.

Firstly, it's essential to recognize that your skin is a part of you, but it does not define you. Everyone's skin is different — it can change with age, fluctuate with hormones, and react to different environments. Accepting this fluidity and appreciating your skin for what it is, rather than lamenting what it is not, can lead to a more positive perception of your self-image.

Embracing your skin also means being gentle and patient with it. It's easy to feel frustrated when skin issues arise, but remember that your skin, like the rest of your body, is a complex system that requires care and understanding. Rather than punishing your skin for its imperfections, respond with kindness and patience. If your skin is experiencing a breakout, treat it gently, provide it with the care it needs, and give it time to heal.

Learning to love your skin also involves reframing the narrative around skincare. Rather than viewing skincare as a means to correct flaws, see it as an act of self-care and nurturing. Use products that make your skin feel good and enjoy the process rather than focusing solely on the results.

Body positivity also applies to skin positivity. In a culture that often glorifies perfection, it's important to celebrate diversity in all its forms, including skin diversity. This includes different skin tones, textures, and conditions. Celebrating this diversity can help reduce stigma and foster a more inclusive, accepting beauty standard.

Loving your skin also involves recognizing and respecting its needs. This means understanding what your skin type is (dry, oily, combination, or sensitive) and using products that suit it. It also means paying attention to how your skin changes with factors like weather, diet, stress, and age, and adapting your skincare routine accordingly.

Embracing your skin as it is doesn't mean ignoring skincare altogether. On the contrary, it's about finding a balance between caring for your skin and accepting its natural state. It's okay to want to improve certain aspects of your skin, but it's important to do so from a place of self-love rather than self-criticism. Remember, skincare is not just about achieving a flawless complexion, it's a journey of understanding, caring for, and ultimately, embracing your skin as it is.